Mastering Homeopathy

Accurate Daily Prescribing for a Successful Practice

Mastering Homeopathy

Accurate Daily Prescribing for a Successful Practice

Jon Gamble
BA, ND, Adv Dip Hom

*K*aruna Publishing

2009

First published in Australia by:
Karuna Publishing
122 Church Street
Wollongong NSW 2500
karuna@bigpond.net.au

©Jon Gamble 2004
Reprinted with corrections 2009

The National Library of Australia
Cataloguing-in-Publication entry:

Gamble, Jon.
>   Mastering homeopathy: accurate daily prescribing for a
>   successful practice.

>   Bibliography.
>   Includes index.
>   ISBN 0 9752473 0 1.

>   1. Homeopathy. I. Title.

>   615.532

Printed by Griffin Press
Cover design by Tina Mulholland

Foreword

The significance of this work by Jon Gamble is best understood by setting it in the context of the present state of the Australian homeopathic community.

During the past decade Australian homeopathy has displayed evidence of becoming a mature profession both administratively and in its practice. The scattered Associations have been able to cooperate in producing a set of National Competencies; a registration body has been created (the Australian Register of Homeopaths); and a large national association of practitioners (the Australian Homeopathic Association) has come into being.

This administrative progress has been more than matched by published work on the practise of homeopathy. Subjects addressed include provings, clinical experience in using some of the proved remedies, miasms, theoretical works and repertories. The standard of much of this work is world class. However, one area that has not been well covered is the relevance of pathology and particular symptoms in daily prescribing.

Anecdotal evidence suggests that many Australian homeopaths tend to see far more chronic cases than acute ones. This is partly a reflection of much of the training provided together with a lack of mentors in acute prescribing. This has certainly been my own experience. A consequence of this situation is to treat particulars as less important than generals or mind symptoms in chronic cases.

However, I was fortunate enough to be invited to participate in the Ear Clinics pioneered by Nyema Hermiston and Patricia Janssen. Here I saw the effectiveness of prescribing when based on an understanding of the pathology of a condition and the accompanying particular symptoms. Results were often rapid and long lasting. The Ear Clinic has now been in existence for almost eight years and has accumulated a valid body of homeopathic clinical evidence in the treatment of chronic ear infections in children.

Jon Gamble participated in the Ear Clinic and also attended some of Dr Parimal Banerji's lectures. These experiences stimulated his thinking about the significance of pathology in chronic cases and its relevance for effective prescribing. This book is the outcome of that thinking.

A major strength of the book is that it provides a theoretical foundation for the results of extended clinical experience. The book rests on a distinction between pathological and functional disturbances. This distinction is clearly explained and appropriate definitions are outlined. A consequence of this distinction is the importance of physical pathology and the relative significance of particulars over generals in its treatment.

A further strength of the book is that Jon has also tested these principles in the treatment of conditions other than chronic children's ear problems. The work provides guidance in treating conditions specific to children, women and men, as well as 30 other diseases not restricted to gender or age. There is also a concise and helpful discussion of posology.

The book is deceptive in that its conciseness tends to conceal the breadth and depth of experience that underpins the discussion of each disease under the headings of *Clinical presentation, Diagnosis & Differential diagnosis, Treatment* and *Summary*. Eight cases are included to demonstrate the application of this and other approaches to treating disease homeopathically.

A perusal of the work of such masters as Boenninghausen, Hering, and Boger reveals the importance of pathology in much of their diagnosis and prescribing. There has been a tendency to ignore this focus. Jon's work is in that tradition and is a contemporary reminder of the significance of pathology for the successful treatment of many diseases. I warmly commend this work to fellow practitioners as a guide and ready work of reference.

John Maitland
BA (Hons) Dip Ed, Adv Dip Hom

Lecturer, Homeopathic History,
Sydney College of Homeopathic Medicine

For Nyema & Rose Li Cai

"The highest ideal of cure is rapid, gentle and permanent restoration of the health..."
(Aphorism 2)

"...the whole array of the symptoms [of a chronic disease] can only be ascertained from the observation of... many single patients affected with such a chronic disease, and without a complete survey and collective picture of these symptoms the medicines capable of curing the whole malady homeopathically... cannot be discovered; and these medicines are, at the same time, the true remedies for the several patients suffering from such chronic affections."
(Aphorism 103)

-- Dr Samuel Hahnemann
The Organon, 5th & 6th ed

"Hypotheses are not to be multiplied beyond necessity"
--William of Occam

CONTENTS

Contents

Preface

While homeopathy achieves remarkable results in ways that no other medicine can, it remains poorly understood and utilised by both the public and the scientific world. The reasons for this may be many, but one of them could be that homeopaths can overlook the everyday aspects of a case. Seeming behavioural difficulties in children may have a pathological cause which might go unnoticed. For example, recurring irritability in children may be caused by delayed teething, low grade ear infection, silent reflux, headache, worms, etc. One may, in choosing a 'mentals' or 'constitutional' prescription, fail to identify factors such as these, which means that the constitutional prescription does not cover such causes.

The therapeutic protocols contained herein are in no way meant to replace the important and demanding work of the constitutional prescription. We have all seen the profound transformation in a patient which the simillimum will produce. The trouble is, our mission in finding that simillimum and giving it in the first consultation can be daunting, incorrect, and often impossible. We can misinterpret complex mentals, or miss an important general which may influence the outcome. In the meantime, the patient, already a little wary about homeopathy, and often coming to us as a last resort after the failure of other therapies, will not gain confidence in either the practitioner or the method. In acute cases, one does not have time to try several different remedies. By that time the patient will already have gone for antibiotics: the first prescription must be a correct one. (I say 'a correct' not 'the correct' because there are many remedies which will improve the case, not just the simillimum).

This book of therapeutic protocols is intended to assist the practitioner to have the patient improving rapidly whilst the practitioner has time to familiarise him/herself with the case and find that constitutional remedy.

No prescriptions in this book are anecdotal, theoretical or in any way removed from the practical realities of treating sick people with homeopathy. All therapeutic recommendations have been used successfully many times over.

I lay this book in the hands of competent and fully trained homeopaths. It is assumed that the reader is familiar with the homeopathic aggravation, the primary and secondary response triggered by a medicine, and Hering's Law of Cure. If the reader is not familiar with these phenomena, it is recommended that the patient is referred to a suitable practitioner. Similarly, one must be familiar with the common symptomatologies of diseases, and the pathological changes which occur with them. A clear diagnosis is essential before following the protocols in this book. As this book is intended only for fully trained homeopaths, it is not to be construed as offering therapeutic advice to lay persons, or practitioners untrained in homeopathy. In such cases, please refer the patient (or yourself) to a homeopath.

J.C.G.
August 2004

Introduction

In 1997 a specialist clinic was established by Nyema Hermiston and Patricia Janssen in Sydney to offer a solution for the epidemic of middle ear diseases which plague children. Middle ear infections are the most common reason a child is taken to the doctor and for which antibiotics are given.

A year later I joined the clinic, then later still, John Maitland. In this clinic we were able to see what homeopathy could do as a front line medicine in the treatment and prevention of ear, nose and throat diseases. However, we also saw that despite what we considered to be accurate constitutional prescribing, some middle ear pathologies remained unchanged. Similarly, looking back over many of my old non-ENT cases, the classical reportorial approach had not yielded an effective remedy. This led me to think that, in order to achieve a good clinical outcome, prescribing which focuses on the particulars (not the generals) of the case is sometimes necessary. We will call this approach, 'pathological prescribing'.

When Is Pathological Prescribing Necessary?

Pathology vs Functional Disturbance
When we treat a sick patient, the illness falls into one of these categories. It is important to decide in which category the illness lies because it will have a bearing on the remedy selection.

Definitions
In this book, a **pathology** is defined as a disease outcome which creates a *long-standing change to the physical structure* of tissues: eg: emphysema. A **functional** disturbance, on the other hand, creates no change to the physical structure: eg: asthma. The only disturbance in asthma is to the *function* of the tissues.

Contention
In my opinion, any remedy can cure a functional disturbance, provided the energetic force of the illness is matched by that remedy. However, where pathological or tissue changes have occurred, due to the chronic disease process, a smaller range of remedies only are able to bring about a cure. A pathology will only be cured by a remedy which is capable of producing the same *physical pathology*. We all practise *Similia*: what a substance can cause it can cure. We wouldn't be homeopaths if we didn't. So we also have to acknowledge the opposite contention: a substance cannot cure what it cannot cause. This is my understanding of why a constitutional remedy may not work when it is used to treat a pathology. For example, you successfully treat a case of asthma with *Ignatia*. Five years later the same patient returns with identical symptoms. However, he is a smoker and since seeing you last time, he has gone on to develop emphysema. Now, even though his symptoms are identical with the

previous presentation, *Ignatia will not be effective*. This is because his functional disturbance has been developed into a pathology. The only effective remedy will be a potentised substance capable of causing emphysema in its crude form. In the first instance you were treating only a functional disturbance. In the second instance, you are now treating a physical pathology.

Empirical evidence
As mentioned, we arrived at this conclusion after observing the large number of cases we had treated of middle ear effusion ('glue ear') in children. Even after good constitutional prescribing and improvement on many levels, some effusions remained unchanged. We needed to prescribe a different remedy to tackle the effusion alone.

The consequence of this contention has a profound effect on remedy selection. It means that when treating a physical pathology, the generals of the patient may become *less* important than the particulars.

This book is not intended to replace competent medical advice, nor should the recommendations be relied upon as representing every possible presentation of illness. The differential diagnoses should not be construed as exhaustive. The therapeutic recommendations are provided as treatment examples which I have used in my clinic. They do not cover every therapeutic possibility.

How to Use this Book

Layout

This book is set out under disease names. Under each disease name, there are the following sub-headings:

- ○ Clinical Presentation
- ○ Diagnosis and Differential Diagnosis
- ○ Treatment
- ○ Summary

Each of these sub-headings is cross referenced throughout the text and index by the paragraph numbers which appear in [square] brackets. The letters "ff" which immediately follow some paragraph number references, refer the reader to the immediately following paragraph numbers.

Some symptoms have been graded according to intensity by the use of '+' signs: with one '+' indicating a minor symptom, and four '+'s indicating a strong one.

The abbreviation 'trit' refers to a powdered trituration.

Appendices
- ○ *Case examples* can be found in Part 5.
- ○ *Practice Forms* are in Part 6.
- ○ *Nutritional and lifestyle handouts* for patients can be found in the Appendices in Part 7. In a busy practice it is easy to forget that nutritional issues may be an obstacle to cure.

Posology

Chronic prescribing
There are of course no fixed rules in regard to posology. The more sensitive the patient is to a medicine, the less they need. If we think a patient is very sensitive, we may give only one dose. For example, in treating a child with violent rages caused by jealousy, *Hyoscyamus 1M* one dose has sufficed. The remedy does not need repetition in such a case unless improvement stalls.

If the remedy is less obvious, or is not close to 'the similimum', we are more likely to repeat it regularly. We may give the remedy once every second, third or fourth day, for one month, before review. We are more likely to adopt this posology, because for many patients, one dose of one remedy is not enough to initiate healing. Patients with long-standing chronic illnesses often need more frequent repetition of the remedy. As a general rule, we repeat potencies of 6, 30 or 200 every second or third day, sometimes for weeks to months. Potencies of

1M we repeat once weekly. We have not found it necessary to succuss, plus or alter the remedy, when using this prescribing method.

Once there is improvement of symptoms, we reduce the frequency of repetition and continue with the same potency. We only increase the potency if the therapeutic value of the remedy starts to wane. For example, a patient who has received a remedy every second day for one or two months, would then be directed to take it every third day for the next month; then every fourth day for the next month, and so on, provided improvement continues.

Where an acute crisis arises during chronic treatment, we postpone chronic treatment whilst treating the acute crisis, and then return to the chronic medicine once the acute has passed. The closer the remedy is to the simillimum, the less likely there will be an acute crisis, or the less severe the acute episode will be.

Acute prescribing

In acute treatment, the more severe the symptom presentation, the more frequent repetition of the remedy is needed, until the symptom severity improves.

Patients are not harmed by repeating medicine often in acute prescribing, provided the frequency of repetition is *either reduced or stopped* upon improvement. If symptoms are improving, reduce the frequency. When symptoms have stopped, stop the remedy.

Potency selection

With each remedy I have given suggested potencies. Whilst potency selection is not indelibly carved in stone, there are reasons for many of the recommended potencies. It was from Dr Parimal Banerji that I first learned that specific potencies are more effective in certain conditions. For example, in treating an otitis media where the tympanum is bright red, *Belladonna 3* is more effective than the higher potencies. *Belladonna 3* is for localised, circumscribed inflammation. *Belladonna 30* is has a greater affinity for the throat, while the 200th is preferred for systemic disease with high fever.

I have adopted the casual approach in describing the centesimal potencies without a letter, eg *Arsenicum 200C* or *200CH* is described as *200*. When a decimal potency is used, it is described as such, eg *200X*.

PART 1: ILLNESSES IN CHILDREN

EAR INFECTIONS & PAINS

[1]
Clinical presentation & Differential diagnosis
To ensure accurate treatment it is essential to inspect the eardrum for colour, contour, transparency and position of the malleus.

Descriptions of middle and external ear diseases are in the categories below. For treatment: see [7] to [15].

[2]
Otitis media (OM)
In otitis media there is pain and sometimes fever. The drum (tympanum) is inflamed and may be pink or red. For treatment see [7].

[3]
Otitis media with effusion (secretory OM)
In otitis media with effusion, as well as the above symptoms, mucus or fluid can often be seen behind the drum which may be bulging. The drum loses its transparency due to fluid in the middle ear. The malleus may be obscured or appear shortened. For treatment see [9].

[4]
Effusion without otitis media (glue ear)
In effusion without otitis media there may be mild pain, or no pain at all. There is no inflammation or fever. Hearing is often impaired, drum motility is reduced or absent, and the drum may be bulging. The light reflexes are distorted or absent.

Drum retraction precedes effusion. In retraction there is no fluid in the middle ear but due to obstructed eustachian tubes (eustachian tube dysfunction), there is negative pressure in the middle ear, resulting in the ear drum being sucked backwards, or beoming retracted.

Both eustachian tube dysfunction, and middle ear effusion, are the most common reasons for the surgical insertion of ventilation tubes (grommets) into the ear drums. For treatment see [11].

[5]
Suppurative otitis media
In suppurative otitis media the drum ruptures, causing a serous, mucous or pussy discharge from the middle ear into the external canal. There may be a little blood which is usually minimal and short-lived. Sometimes all that the parents note is a small dried spot of mucus on the child's pillow.

Drum rupture following otitis media with effusion is nature's way of expelling the purulent matter from the middle ear. Once the rupture has taken place, the healthy drum will repair itself within a few days. During that time, absolutely no water must be allowed to enter the ear canal. In rare cases, particularly if there have been multiple drum ruptures or repeated sets of ventilation tubes (grommets) inserted, the drum will not heal. These cases are usually left untreated until the child is 10 year's old and can undergo reconstructive surgery. While homeopathy is able to help some, surgery is needed for many cases. For treatment see [13].

[6]
Chronic otitis externa (swimmer's ear)
There is a chronic, purulent, sometimes smelly, discharge in the external ear canal. The drum is intact, and there may be an opaque film covering it. The patient may experience tenderness, but more often no pain at all. There may be itching. Frequently the only symptom is a recurring, annoying discharge. For treatment see [15].

Treatment
Treatment is divided into these categories:
- [7] Otitis media
- [9] Otitis media with effusion
- [11] Effusion without otitis media
- [12] Deafness
- [13] Suppurative otitis media (drum rupture)
- [14] Chronic or repetitive otitis media
- [15] Chronic otitis externa (swimmer's ear)

[7]
Otitis media
- *Ferrum phos 200:* Mid-range fever with red cheeks, some pain, the drum is pink to red.
- *Belladonna 3:* Mid to high fever with flushing and red drum, some pain and rapid onset. If there is no fever but the drum is red, *Belladonna 3* is still effective.

Belladonna and *Ferrum phos* are the most common remedies needed for acute otitis media. In other cases, the following are needed:
- *Aconite 4x:* Mid-range or high fever, some redness of drum and face but less than *Belladonna*, and with anxiety, *restlessness* and pain. Indicated also after exposure to cold winds.
- *Arsenicum 3:* Pain+++ with anxiety and night aggravation, especially where other remedies fail.
- *Chamomilla 30:* Pain+++ with irritability or ear pain with or without inflammation associated with dentition.
- *Kreosotum 200:* If *Chamomilla* fails.
- *Coffea 200:* If there is also sleep disturbance, especially during teething.

- *Hepar sulph 200:* Pain++ with sore submandibular glands associated with pharyngitis or tonsillitis.

As otitis media is an acute situation, it may be necessary to alternate the above remedies: eg, a red drum occurring during teething often needs *Belladonna 3* alternating with *Chamomilla 30* for a rapid result.

[8]
Summary

- *Belladonna 3:* Red drum.
- *Ferrum phos 200:* Pink drum.
- *Hepar sulph 200:* Ear pain from tonsillitis.
- *Chamomilla 30*: Ear pain with teething.
- *Aconite* 4x: Ear pain after exposure to cold wind + restlessness.
- *Arsenicum 3:* Ear pain unresponsive to other remedies.

[9]
Otitis media with effusion

- If the drum is **red**, begin with *Belladonna 3* until the drum is no longer red (one or two days in most cases) then switch to *Kali mur 3x mixed with Ferrum phos 3x trit*. These come in powders and may be mixed into menstruum and succussed, giving a 4x potency, which is just as effective as the fresh powder. Give at least three times daily, or half hourly to two hourly if there is pain.
- If the drum is **pink** with a *low to medium* range fever, use *Ferrum phos 200* until the fever has gone, then change to *Ferrum phos/Kali mur 3x*, as described above.
- Once the inflammatory stage has passed, and there is only an effusion remaining (ie no sign of drum inflammation or fever), change to *Pulsatilla 30* mixed with *Kali mur 3x trit*. (Adding of *Kali mur* powder seems to potentiate the action of the *Pulsatilla*.) If there is pain, give this three times daily, reducing upon improvement. Continue daily when the pain has cleared, to clear remaining mucus from the middle ear and eustachian tubes. This usually takes one to four weeks.
- *Aconite* and *Arsenicum* can be used in the situations described under Otitis Media at [7].

[10]
Summary

- Effusion with pink drum and low-medium fever: Start with *Ferrum phos 200*, then *Ferrum phos 3x mixed with Kali mur 3x*, repeated half hourly.
- *Belladonna 3:* Fever, pain, red drum.
- *Pulsatilla 30 mixed with Kali mur 3x:* No fever, no inflamed drum, but effusion and slight pain or no pain.

[11]
Effusion without otitis media
- *Pulsatilla 30:* Effusion with bulging drum but no inflammation: start with *Pulsatilla 30* or *200*, mixed with *Kali mur 3x* as described above. If it is a chronic problem, continue this mix once daily for a month. This is also the remedy of choice for eustachian tube dysfunction.
- *Ferrum phos 200:* If the drum is pink and the child has a fever, give *Ferrum phos 200*. If there is only a hint of fever or slight pinkness of the drum, give *Ferrum phos/Kali mur 3x* mixed as described above.
- *Kali mur 3x:* Effusion with a white-coated tongue and signs of lymphatic congestion: *Kali mur 3x* or *4x* three times daily plus a dairy free diet.
- If the above measures are unsuccessful: give *Tuberculinum bov 1M*, which can bring a quick result. In some cases one dose will suffice.

If there is any sign of lymphatic congestion (eg lymph rosary in the iris) cow's milk products should be removed from the diet. In some cases, dietary modification alone can clear an effusion, but the result is hastened by the use of the above medicines.

In typical cases we now use the following protocol to remove middle ear effusion in young children: One dose of *Tuberculinum bov 1M* at time of consultation, then follow the next day with one dose daily of *Pulsatilla 30 mixed with Kali mur 3x*. Continue this for four weeks. Provided there is good improvement at second visit, maintain the dietary regimes if given, and reduce the *Pulsatilla/Kali mur* mix to one dose every second day.

For children four years and older the use of Otovents (nose balloons) are very useful in mechanically opening eustachian tubes. The child occludes one nostril with their finger while blowing up the nose balloon with the other nostril, then swallowing: this can open the eustachian tubes.

If the above protocol has not yielded a result by the second visit: try excluding all milk, reduce wheat and identify one of the following causes:

1. **Vaccinosis**: See the discussion at [33].
2. **Adenoid enlargement**: Look for snoring or mouth breathing. Hypertrophy of the adenoids can be a result of persistent low grade inflammation, which may have an allergic aetiology. Thus it is important to identify any food allergies (or sensitivities) and withdraw them. If there are signs of inflammation in the nasal passages, give *Ferrum phos/Kali mur 3x* mix twice daily and *Baryta carb* 200 every second day. If there are no signs of inflammation or allergy, give *Baryta-carb* 200 alone. Enlarged adenoids can also respond to *Calcarea carb, Lachesis, Silicea, Thuja* and *Tuberculinum*.
3. **Intestinal parasites**: Look for symptoms such as: umbilical pain, night terrors, nasal or rectal itch, variable appetite and variable bowel habits. Give either of these remedies:
   - *Nux vom 30 alternating with Stannum met 200* if abdominal pain is the key symptom; or

- *Cina 200* if rectal itch and aggressive behaviour are uppermost. See [25].
4. **Miasmatic**: The following remedies are capable of resolving a middle ear effusion:
   - *Tuberculinum 1M:* (Multiple airborne allergies- especially to cat fur.)
   - *Silicea 30/200:* (Sensitivity to cold, shyness, chronicity, fine boned.)
   - *Medorrhinum 200:* (Sleep position; genito-urinary symptoms; refuses to go to bed; sycotic family history.)
   - *Lycopodium 200:* (Variable bowel habits with flatulence; bossy at home but timid at school; 4pm aggravation; hypoglycaemic irritability.)
   - *Carcinosin 30/200:* (Fastidious; family history of cancer; affected by the seaside.)
   - *Phosphorus 30/200:* (Over-sensitive; bright; fears dark, storms: ailments go quickly into the chest.)
   - *Calcarea carb 30:* (Happy to play alone; nocturnal head sweats; huge appetite; strong willed but placid.)
   - *Psorinum 1M:* Beneficial when used between attacks, or after resolving a case of effusion, to prevent relapse.
   - *Mercurius 200:* Pain is severe, at night.

While this list of remedies is not exhaustive, bear in mind that middle ear effusion is a physical pathology. A constitutional medicine may improve a child's general characteristics, but unless it is capable of causing effusion in crude form, it may not resolve the problem.

5. **Stubborn effusions**. We have also resolved stubborn effusions with *Pulsatilla 30* mixed with *Pyrogenium 200* in the same bottle, given regularly for two to three weeks. This is particularly useful if the colour of the effusion is yellow or very dense: ie a purulent fluid.

Notes
1. *Allergy*: Clinical signs: dark circles under eyes; inflammation of nasal passages
2. *Lymphatic congestion*: White coated tongue; iris signs (eg lymph rosary)
3. *Nutrition*: Check about sound nutrition. Look for white spots on fingernails, restless extremeties or mouth ulcers (zinc deficiency). See the nutritional information under Part 7: Appendices.

[12]
Deafness *(see discussion of effusion above)*
Where the cause is catarrh, *Pulsatilla* and *Kali mur* mix can be used (see above). If there has been a history of drum perforation, these medicines work better in some cases:
- *Kali sulph 30:* The discharge was watery.
- *Kali bich 30*: The discharge was thick or stringy.
However, it is recommended that treatment starts with *Pulsatilla 30/Kali mur 3x mix*, which often gives the best result.
 In stubborn cases:

- *Tuberculinum bov 1M:* One or two doses.
- DPT/Pedvax or occasionally Hepatitis B vaccine in potency: See Vaccinosis at [33]. (If the child was given the new DTPa it is better to use this. If unsure, we mix both DPT and DTPa together.)
- Combine homeopathic treatment with twice daily used of Otovents.

[13]
Drum rupture (suppurative otitis media)
- *Pulsatilla 30 or 200:* Facilitates healing of the drum and absorbs the fluid. Stop the medicine once the drum has granulated. It may be continued in the presence of any remaining effusion.
- *Silicea 200:* In an old perforation which is not healing, try *Silicea 200* every second day.
- *Mercurius 200:* for chronic cases where symptoms come on at night.

[14]
Chronic or repetitive otitis media
The above remedies may be used both acutely and chronically, repeated at regular intervals. However one of the following medicines may be needed to cure the case, depending on symptoms: *Sulphur 200; Psorinum 1M; Tuberculinum bov 1M.* These should be given between attacks. Also consider other miasmatic remedies, as mentioned above.

We know that DPT (and DTPa) vaccination causes ENT pathologies in some children, so this can be used as a remedy for stubborn glue ear and infection (regardless as to whether the child had a reaction to the said vaccine). In Australia, because the DTPa is now mixed with Pedvax, we give both mixed as one remedy. See the protocol at [34] for using vaccines in potency.

A well indicated constitutional medicine may *not* resolve a middle ear effusion. (The list given above shows constitutional remedies which have been shown as capable of resolving effusion.) See the discussion in the introduction concerning the treatment of pathologies vs functional disturbances.

[15]
Chronic otitis externa or swimmer's ear
Chronic swimmer's ear or otitis externa can be a fungal or bacterial infection or both, and can persist in adults for decades without significant improvement. It is highly resistant to treatment. However, it can respond steadily to homeopathy. Water must be strictly excluded from the ear until cured.

It is often assumed that a chronic otitis externa is fungal in origin. We know from experience that this is not always the case. The only way to really be sure is to have a swab from the ear cultured. Armed with a pathology report, one is then able to choose an isopathic prescription which can be given in both oral and aural drops. However, we have still succeeded in curing otitis externa without specific cultures, by giving the oral and ear drops below:

Oral drops: *Pseudomonas + Aspergillus + Golden staph* all mixed together + either *Silicea, Hepar sulph, or Graphites*, in ascending potencies starting from 200.

Ear drops: same as above, minus the *Silicea*, in pure ethanol for adults; or if a child, prepare the medicine in a mix of either brandy or hydrogen peroxide, with a 50 per cent distilled water added.

Choosing Silicea 200, Hepar sulph 200 or Graphites 200:

- *Silicea:* Persistence or stubbornness of complaints; poor healing ability; long history of outer ear conditions without any other fungal or infective complaint. Cold aggravation. History of tympanum rupture.
- *Hepar sulph*: Pain; swollen sub-mandibular glands; history of throat and ear infections.
- *Graphites:* History of fungal infections, eg tinea.

Dosage instructions:

- Repeat every other day for at least one month before moving up in potency.
- At the same time, the patient alternates the **ear** drops in a base or either pure ethanol (adult), brandy or hydrogen peroxide (child).
- Use *Psorinum 1M* as an intercurrent, weekly.
- **Caution**: do not give pure ethanol if there is inflammation evident in the ear canal. Do not give any ear drops in the presence of drum perforation.

The oral and ear drops should be given on alternate days in ascending potencies over many months. Abstaining from sugar and yeast in the diet during treatment can yield a better result.

All water (including salt water) must be kept out of the ear canal until all symptoms have been removed.

Summary
Month 1
- **Oral drops:** Identified organism **or** above triad mix in potency + *Silicea 200* mixed: every second day (three times per week)
- **Ear drops**: As above minus the *Silicea (or Graphites or Hepar sulph)* (dispensed in pure ethanol or peroxide) every second day.
- *Psorinum 1M:* one dose per week (on the day when not taking the above).

Month 2
- **Oral drops**: same as for month one, increased in potency to 1M + *Silicea 200* mixed: every other day.
- **Ear drops:** Same as for month one now in 1M potency
- *Psorinum 1M* weekly.

Continue monthly, raising potency of the fungi/bacteria to 10M, 50M etc, plus the *Silicea 200* (not raised in potency) until cured.

For a case example, see Part 5, Case 6.

TONSILLITIS, LARYNGITIS & PHARYNGITIS

[16]
Clinical presentation
These three diseases of the throat are included together, since the remedies are similar for each, and the clinical presentation may include more than one illness at once. The colour and size of the tissues help to refine the prescription, so be sure to inspect the tonsils and surrounding tissues, as well as taking the subjective symptoms.

Common symptoms are:

Tonsillitis
- o Inflammation – bright or dusky etc
- o Enlargement of tonsils, sometimes with white spots
- o Fever (high fever if streptococcal tonsillitis)
- o Slight to severe pain
- o Slight cough
- o Cervical glands enlarged, sometimes tender.

Pharyngitis
- o Inflammation or congestion, mottled or dimpled redness at posterior wall of pharynx behind the tonsils, sometimes small red spots
- o Slight pain
- o Slight cough
- o If there is a stridor, it is likely to be croup – not pharyngitis.

Laryngitis
- o Laryngeal pain
- o Hoarse voice or aphonia
- o Cough – usually productive.

[17]
Treatment
Hepar sulph 200 is the main remedy for tonsillitis, pharyngitis and laryngitis. It covers up to 75% of cases: tonsillitis without pus, throat cough, and painful cervical glands, an inflamed pharynx, hoarse voice or aphonia.

Always ask the patient, which symptom is worrying him/her the most. Then use this symptom as the starting point for the prescription.

This section is divided into these categories:
- o *[18] Tonsillitis*
- o *[19] Laryngitis*
- o *[20] Pharyngitis*

[18]
Tonsillitis
- *Hepar sulph 200:* The main remedy for tonsillitis, as described above.

Other remedies:
- *Mercurius* group remedies: Where *pain in the glandular tissue* is the main focus, one of the mercuries is usually necessary. Pain is sharp and may radiate from the cervical glands to the ear: if left sided give *Mercurius iod rub 200*; if right sided give *Mercurius iod flav 200*.
- *Phytolacca 200:* If the tissue surrounding the tonsils is inflamed, and there is sharp pain radiating to the ear. The patient may already have tried antibiotics, which are often ineffective with this type of pain.
- *Mercurius cyanatus 200*: If there is severe pain with **dysphagia, high fever and septic white patches** (usually streptococcal), give *Mercurius cy 200*. This prescription works more rapidly than antibiotics.

[19]
Laryngitis
- *Hepar sulph 200*: The medicine *par excellence*. Hoarse voice, sore glands, and perhaps a throat cough.

Other remedies:
- *Arum triph 30*: Hoarseness or bitonal voice with severe burning laryngeal pain.
- *Causticum 200*: Loss of voice, tickling in larynx, and constant desire to swallow.
- *Phosphorus 200*: The larynx is painful with tickling and loss of voice worse in the evening or cold air. Symptoms proceed rapidly to the throat (in a matter of one or two hours).

All the above remedies for laryngitis should be thought of whenever there is loss of voice (aphonia).
- *Phytolacca 200:* Pain is felt in the glands and may radiate to the ears.
- *Argentum met 200:* Loss of voice, especially from overuse. Raw pain on coughing which is aggravated by laughing or talking.

[20]
Pharyngitis
- *Hepar sulph 200*: Again the main medicine. Sore throat, low fever, dry cough, tender cervical glands.

Other remedies:
- *Phytolacca 200*: In a small number of cases not only the posterior wall of the pharynx, but the tissue *surrounding* the tonsils is inflamed. There may be sharp pain in the glands, which may radiate to the ears.
- *Causticum, Phosphorus & Arum triph,* as described in [19].

If the tonsils are affected, see [18].

CROUP & OTHER COUGHS

[21]
Clinical presentation for croup
o Sudden onset
o Dyspnoea due to inflammation of the trachea or larynx
o Laryngeal stridor on inspiration
o Possible cyanosis if severe
o Characteristic hoarse, barking cough
o Anxiety
o Onset in cold weather.

[22]
Treatment
Croup: Sub-acute
- *Bromium 6*: Practitioners are more likely to see the child the morning after an episode of croup the previous night and there is still croupy cough and stridor persisting. In this sub-acute stage give *Bromium 6* every two hours until bedtime, repeating at night if the child is woken by the croup.

Croup: Acute
If the croup is in its acute, severe stage (usually at night), with dyspnoea, loud stridor and distress:
- *Bromium 1M*: one dose will often suffice.

Other remedies:
- *Spongia 30*: Sibilant sound as though a saw is driven through wood.
- *Hepar sulph 200: Loose* croupy cough.
- *Moschus 200:* Great anxiety (works better than *Aconite* owing to *Moschus'* affinity with the throat).

Caution: If the child (1) can only breathe through the mouth; (2) *must* sit up; (3) has a stridor on expiration **and** inspiration, the likely diagnosis is: **epiglottitis**. This is a rare but life-threatening illness which should be referred immediately for emergency care. Do not under any circumstances use a tongue depressor in the presence of these symptoms.

Non-croupy cough in infants (including bronchiolitis):
- *Ipecac 30*: Loose and rattly cough in children, such as in bronchiolitis, *Ipecac* gives the most consistent results, even if there is no vomiting. See the chart of symptom differentials at [81].
- *Antimony tart 30*: The child is distressed *and unable to take* a proper breath (not common in bronchiolitis), *Antimony tart 30* may work better than *Ipecac* in these circumstances.

[23]
General cough remedies (adults & children)

Here are some other indicators for cough remedies:

- *Cuprum met 6*: Spasmodic cough.
- *Hepar sulph 200*: The main remedy for a throat cough, particularly where the submandibular glands are swollen, or with a sore throat.
- *Spongia 30*: Sibilant, dry cough which has a 'sawing' sound. Aggravation from bending the head backwards. Burning sensation in the larynx. The *Spongia* cough is sometimes better by eating.
- *Hyoscyamus 6*: One of the best remedies for a cough which mainly occurs at night, waking the patient from sleep. Especially effective in children.
- *Bryonia 30 or 200*: Cough with chest pain, worse in warm room. Head pain during the cough (patient holds head while coughing).
- *Causticum 30 or 200*: The cough is so deep s/he cannot seem to reach deeply enough to expectorate the phlegm. Aggravation from bending head forwards.
- *Rumex 30:* Dry tickle in throat provokes the cough which is worse from inspiring cool air and at night. Includes sudden changes in air temperature, such as when undressing at night.
- *Sanguinaria 200*: Any cough which occurs with burping, or is better with passing flatus.
- *Kreosotum 200*: Cough from changing position in bed.
- *Drosera 30*: For spasmodic night cough. Patient holds the abdomen during the cough.
- *Phosphorus 30 or 200*: The cough has *moved rapidly* into the chest (cf *Kali iod*). The cough may be worse from strong odours.
- *Conium 3 or 6*: There is a small, dry spot in the larynx producing the cough.
- *Antimony tart 30*: Cough from sun exposure. Loud rattling cough with chest phlegm which cannot be expectorated.
- *Natrum carb 200*: Cough comes on in the summer heat.
- *Coccus cacti 6*: Persistent, sometimes suffocative paroxysms of coughing which originate from a tickle in the throat, and conclude in expectorating or vomiting thick mucus.

See also the discussion of asthma and chronic obstructive pulmonary disease at [80] ff.

ABDOMINAL PAIN IN CHILDREN

[24]
Differential diagnosis &
Treatment
The conditions described in this section can all cause abdominal pain in children. For a summary of differential diagnoses and relevant questions to ask about unsettled babies: see [32].

[25]
Intestinal parasites
The most common cause of abdominal pain in children that we are likely to see is intestinal parasites. There are a variety of such parasites, apart from common worms. Proper hygiene, especially where pets are kept in the house, is important. However, a child who is constitutionally susceptible will easily contract parasitic infection, despite good hygiene.

Confirmatory signs of intestinal parasites are: teeth grinding during sleep; unexplained night terrors; nasal or rectal itch; unexplained temper tantrums or aggressive behaviour and variable appetite.

The remedy selection is still based on the presenting symptomatology, regardless of which parasite is present.
- *Nux vom 30 alternating with Stannum met 200:* Where there is abdominal pain which is experienced around the umbilicus: give *Nux vom 30* one day alternating with *Stannum met 200:* alternate days for one to two months.
- *Cina 200:* Where there is no umbilical pain, but rectal or nasal itch and irritability, give *Cina 200* on alternate days for at least one month.

Many children with unexplained aggressive behaviour respond positively to either of the above two protocols for parasite elimination.
Note that intestinal parasites occur in adults as well as children, though this goes largely undiagnosed. See Irritable Bowel Syndrome at [148]. For more detail on this topic see Gamble, J, *Mastering Homeopathy 2: The Treatment of Irritable Bowel Syndrome* (2006).

[26]
Uretal reflux
A surprising number of cases of persistent crying have turned out to be uretal reflux or cystitis. In uretal reflux there may be no symptoms at all, yet the crying will always stop once a course of antibiotics is given. This will lead the doctor to presume the problem was an ear infection. However evidence can only be found with analysis of the baby's urine. Most cases respond well to *Cantharis 200*. If *Cantharis* does not work, try *Medorrhinum 1M*. Referral for medical assessment is essential since in some cases there is possibility of renal damage.

[27]
Anxiety
Another common cause of abdominal pain is anxiety. If the child manifests the abdominal pain before going to school, but seldom on the weekends, then anxiety is the likely cause. *Silicea, Phosphorus, Opium,* and *Ignatia* are the most common remedies we have used. See Anxiety at [183].

[28]
Constipation
Carefully check the details of the child's exact bowel habits.
- *Nux vom 30:* If the bowels do not completely evacuate, there is incomplete peristalsis, which can result in abdominal pain. A child who sits for a long time on the toilet, yet passes little stool for all the effort, is likely to be in this category. *Nux vom 30,* repeated every second day, will often correct the problem.
- *Bryonia 200:* Where the child passes no stool for several days, then passes a large, hard stool, and nausea or pain is more likely felt in the upper abdominal region. *Bryonia* has cured many cases of this type of stubborn constipation in children and adults.
- *Thuja 6:* Where the child is frightened to pass a stool owing to a history of sphincter trauma or pain, *Thuja 6* can cure. If *Thuja* fails, consider *Calcarea carb 30.*
- *Alumina 200:* If the stool is very soft, is passed with difficulty or only every few days.
- *Nitric ac 200:* The child stiffens up or winces when the stool starts to pass. There may be a smear of blood. Either of these may be a sing of anal fissure in children. This remedy is specific for anal fissure.

[29]
Appendicitis
Abdominal pain with fever but no diarrhoea is a red bullet symptom for appendicitis. If the rebound test is positive and there is clear right abdominal tenderness with guarding, these are good confirming points. Referral for medical care is advised if symptoms become more severe.

- If in its early stages, most cases of appendicitis will respond to *Lycopodium 30* alternating with *Belladonna 30* one to two hourly until improvement, then on alternate days until the patient is fully recovered.

[30] Colic
Symptoms are flatulence, tympanic abdomen and pain.
- *Lycopodium 30 or 200:* If the colic occurs a long time after feeding. Check there is no constipation.
- *Morgan Pure 30:* In obstinate colic, unresponsive to the usual remedies, we have found the bowel nosode *Morgan Pure* has saved the day. For more information see Colic at [41] and Reflux at [40].

There may be food sensitivity in cases of obstinate colic in babies, in which case the mother should abstain from those foods. The most common food sensitivities are: wheat, egg, dairy, yeast and salicylates.

[31]
Pyloric stenosis
There is projectile vomiting after feeding.
- *Aethusa 200:* The main remedy in pyloric stenosis. Also use in cases where there is no pyloric stenosis, yet the child clearly reacts to breast milk, with colic or indigestion. This should be repeated every 2nd day for many weeks.
- *Dysentery Co 30:* Use this bowel nosode if *Aethusa* fails. According to Foubister it is a specific for pyloric stenosis, yet we have found that *Aethusa* rarely fails.

[32]
Summary of Differential diagnosis
Intestinal parasites: teeth grinding, rectal or nasal itch, night terrors, unexplained irritability, appetite changes.
Uretal reflux and cystitis: check for urinary symptoms.
Anxiety: there is a relationship between the pain and certain events.
Constipation: Check the child's exact bowel habits. Even though a child may sit on the toilet each day there may be incomplete evacuation.
Appendicitis: observe abdominal reflux response: suspect appendicitis if it is positive, and especially if there is a fever and appetite loss.
Colic: flatulence, abdominal gurgling, pain.
Pyloric stenosis: projectile vomiting after feeding.

Questions to ask when babies are unsettled:
- o How often is a stool passed? (Constipation?)
- o Is the pain related to feeding, if so does it come on soon or a long time after?
- o Is there a fever? (Infection likely)
- o Is there much flatulence or belching? (Colic or reflux)
- o Do you hear much gurgling and rumbling in the abdomen? (Colic)
- o Is there a family history of food intolerances?
- o Is there vomiting after feeding? (Possibly pyloric stenosis.)

Additional questions for older children:
- o Where exactly is the abdominal pain? (Umbilical pain suggests parasites)
- o Is there rectal itch?
- o Is there a relationship between the pain and certain events or certain times of the day? (suggestive of anxiety)

VACCINOSIS

Overview

Vaccinosis, first recognised by Burnett in the early 20th century, remains a common phenomenon in the 21st century. Whilst it is advisable to take preventative disease care, the problem is that there are so many more vaccines given now than in Burnett's day. This has resulted in the phenomenon of 'Vaccinosis' becoming more widespread.

The number of vaccinations in the Australian Immunisation Schedule has increased at an alarming rate, with dubious consideration and little research given to the long term impact on child health. There appears to be no careful thought given to actual disease risks, compared to the consequences of the variety of chemicals and biological materials being injected into babies. Neither the medical nor the homeopathic community know what the long term effects of this are on the developing immune system. There is now a real concern that 'stealth' viruses are being introduced into the human environment from viruses formerly associated with animals. See the discussion of Chronic Fatigue Syndrome at [125] ff.

There is also growing debate about whether the antibody response triggered by vaccination, is sufficient to generate a complete immune response.

In Australia, a child is given the hepatitis B vaccine *at birth*, two, four and six months. The usual ways to contract this disease are through unprotected intercourse or illicit drug use, activities that only an extraordinarily adventurous newborn would undertake. In the early 1990s, when the hepatitis B vaccination was first promoted for use in children, the manufacturer was reprimanded by the pharmaceutical industry body for overstating the case for the need for hepatitis B in children!

At age two months, children receive vaccinations for whooping cough, diphtheria, tetanus, polio and haemophilus influenzae B and hepatitis B *at the same time!* This is repeated at four and six months and on it goes. Any child who is sensitive either to the additives or pathogens in the vaccine, can have long term sequelae. The advent of these sequelae are generally denied or unrecognised by the medical profession.

We have noted that the children most at risk from vaccination have a strong family history of allergy.

Somewhere between 10 to 20 per cent of children have, in our estimation, some form of long term sequelae from vaccination. This hypothesis is confirmed when the vaccine is prescribed in potency and the symptoms improve. If anyone wishes to describe a child's chronic health problems which are corrected after homeopathically neutralising the side effects of vaccination, as 'anecdotal', then let us all have anecdotal practices: the result will be healthier children.

Our observation is that by far the most problematic of the vaccines was the DPT and DTPa. The most common sequelae was respiratory illness. The new Pedvax does not appear to cause these respiratory symptoms, yet its introduction is still too recent to clinically assess long term trends. Thankfully, all vaccines since 2000 are mercury-free. Most of vaccine side effects concern the respiratory system: typically upper respiratory infections and catarrh. With the DPT many children went on to develop stubborn middle ear effusion and otitis media, which will not resolve with the usual remedies until the vaccine is given in potency. Other children will develop asthma or bronchiolitis. Still others have their predisposed allergic sensitivities increased after vaccination. More obscure symptoms can be insomnia and behavioural disturbances such as unprovoked temper tantrums; inability to attach to the parents (including autistic spectrum disorder); headaches; nightmares and abdominal pain. We are convinced that sub-clinical encephalopathy occurs in some cases. In other cases, many months after receiving a vaccine, an unexplained high fever (including fitting) can occur.

Often behavioural disturbances occur with various kinds of bowel disturbance, which may include smelly flatulence, food intolerances, unformed stools, or other syndromes often described as 'leaky gut' or dysbiosis.

When we see a grouping of the symptoms listed below, we consider it as a *prima facie* case of DPT (or DTPa) vaccinosis:
o Frequent waking
o Nocturnal fevers
o Repeated otitis media &/or middle ear effusion
o Repeated coughs, colds, wheezes
o Weight loss
o Aggravation from DPT/Pedvax vaccination (eg persistent or high fever)
o Symptoms began shortly after vaccination
o Head-banging.
When suspecting vaccinosis, important points are:
o Was there a high or persistent fever after the vaccine?
o Was there a persistent lump at the site of the injection?
o Did the child's illness begin shortly after a vaccination?

After DPT, the MMR seems to cause similar problems. Readers will be aware of Dr Wakefield's research which examined an alleged link between MMR and autism, especially in males. There is a wide body of anecdotal evidence which give weight to this contention.

We have also identified cases where we believe Hepatitis B is a causative factor in vaccinosis.

The new *Gardisil* vaccination for HPV is quickly becoming the most notorious. In a number of our patients we have seen strange neurological disturbances, and there have been documented cases of post inoculation Guillian-Barré syndrome.

[34]
Treatment
Vaccinosis treatment regime
We use the vaccinosis antidoting protocols derived from the works of Drs Tinus Smits and Jean Elmiger. The original vaccine material is potentised and given to the patient in scaled potencies as described below. With the modern vaccine program, insidious iatrogenic disease is prevalent to a degree never before seen.

Where there were clear symptoms after a vaccination (such as a fever), those symptoms will often return once the vaccine is given in potency. This fever, or indeed any symptoms arising from administration of the potentised vaccine, should not be interfered with. Symptoms will in most cases run their course without intervention within 24 hours.

If possible, give the potentised vaccine in *at least* three repeated doses of 30, 200 and 1M. We normally give one dose per day for 5 to 10 days of each potency in ascending order. For example:

- 1. *Hexa 30* once daily for 5 days.
- 2. *Hexa 200* once daily for 5 days.
- 3. *Hexa 1M* once daily for 5 days.
- Stop the regime if an aggravation occurs, then resume and continue administration of that potency until there are no further aggravations. We find that repeated doses of the 30th and 200th potencies usually suffice.

Summary
- *Vaccine mix 30*: one dose daily for 5 to 10 days. Stop if there is an aggravation; wait for the aggravation to pass, and then resume. When no more aggravation or effect, go up to next potency:
- *Vaccine mix 200*: same dose as above. If no aggravation or effect, treatment is concluded. If there is aggravation or effect, go up to the next potency:
- *Vaccine mix 1M*: same dose as above.

Practitioners are referred to the work of Dr Tinus Smits for elaboration. See the Bibliography.

The history and symptoms can be so confused that it is impossible to know where to start. Apart from the vaccination schedule, the child may have had multiple courses of antibiotics, plus cortico-steroids, Ventolin or Seretide. You suspect that the child's disease is iatrogenic, but where do you start? In these cases, begin treatment with *Camphor 200*, two doses daily for up to a week (or longer if there is long-term use of cortico-steroids). This often clears the case well so that a second remedy choice becomes more reliable. We have also found in cases of unexplained intermittent fevers (which are not always vaccination induced) *Camphor 200* can cure.

Another approach favoured by many homeopaths is to give the constitutional medicine for the patient. In some cases this is all that may be required, in others vaccinosis can remain as an obstacle to cure.

See the discussion of gut problems [38] and the use of bowel nosodes at [127].

HOMEOPROPHYLAXIS

[35]
Overview
Whilst homeoprophylaxis is not a disease, we have placed it here because it has a role in disease prevention (not treatment).

Parents requesting homeoprophylaxis should both attend for a consultation so that there is ample opportunity to discuss the implications of homeoprophylaxis. It is not appropriate to prescribe homeoprophylaxis without a consultation. It is important to support the parents' decision about vaccination, whilst answering questions accurately and without bias.

[36]
Parents decide to give orthodox vaccination
In this situation, we recommend administration of the potentised vaccine in the 30th or 200th potency, just prior and following the respective vaccination. It can be given daily for three days after the vaccination. This can minimise the likelihood of post-vaccination sequelae (vaccinosis).

[37]
Parents decide to use homeoprophylaxis
Practitioners should be aware that homeoprophylaxis entails giving nosodes, ***not potentised vaccine material***. The latter is only used to treat the side-effects caused by a specific vaccination. See [33].

The greatest efficacy in homeoprophylaxis is likely to be achieved if the nosode is given during an outbreak of the relevant disease. This is certainly the experience of Dorothy Sheppard in the prevention of whooping cough. Nonetheless, as recommended by Isaac Golden, parents often prefer to have a schedule they can follow. The reader is referred to Mr Golden's pioneering research and recommended prophylaxis protocol. See the Bibliography.

Our own view is that one is wise to take precautions against potentially dangerous diseases *to which the child is likely to be exposed.* Whooping cough and measles can be very serious in infants, and both still occur in isolated outbreaks in Australia. If the mother has had measles, the child is more likely to be protected from that disease for as long as breast feeding continues. Children in Australia are unlikely to be exposed to diseases such as diphtheria, hepatitis B, and polio. However, it is sensible to take precautions against likely circumstances: for example, prophylaxis for tetanus in older children. See also the work of Dr Tinus Smits in the Bibliography.

It is equally sensible not to inflict multiple vaccines (or unnecessary homeopathic remedies) on infant immune systems for disease events which are unlikely to occur.

Whilst we can use specific disease-prevention measures, it is easy to forget, in the current fear-driven climate, that immunity is maximised by breast feeding, good nutrition and a nurturing home environment.

We also need to be aware of these factors:

- o Individuals have susceptibility to certain types of diseases
- o Individuals with allergic backgrounds may have reactions to vaccination and special needs therefore need to be addressed
- o Public health authorities do not acknowledge the efficacy of homeoprophylaxis
- o Orthodox vaccination is not compulsory for school admission in Australia (despite a common perception to the contrary)
- o All advice, recommendations and discussion with clients on homeoprophylaxis should be carefully recorded.

Please see the recommended forms and schedules in regard to homeoprophylaxis in Part 6. One should also note the homeoprophylaxis statement issued by the Australian Register of Homeopaths for practitioners, which can be viewed at www.aroh.com.au

BEHAVIOURAL PROBLEMS IN CHILDREN RELATED TO GUT FUNCTION

[38]
Overview

The relationship between gut and brain function is becoming increasingly more recognised. Clinically, we have certainly noted this relationship.

The gut contains neuro-transmitters which also form a large part of immune system activity. Many health authorities, including WHO, recommend that wheat and especially dairy should not be introduced before 12 months of age, due to the immaturity of the gut. When one considers how many children have been introduced to these foods, as well as drugs such as antibiotics, before their digestive systems are mature enough, the reasons for gut problems become apparent. Children with a family history of food sensitivity or allergies are more susceptible. Gut dysfunction affects the absorption of nutrients, including zinc, which has a crucial affect on the immune system.

The widespread and often indiscriminate use of antibiotics which has arisen since the 1960s, both as prescriptions from the doctor and agriculturally in our food chain, continues to cause the successive diminution if the quality of gut flora from one generation to the next. The newborn child enters the world with already compromised gut flora inherited from the compromised gut flora of the parents. Add a course of two of antibiotics, ever more frequently given to mothers prior to labour as prevention against streptococcus B, and the flora is further diminished, resulting in gut dysbiosis. Here is the ground from which grows the wide spectrum of food sensitivity and food allergy, which is increasingly more common with each generation.

[39]
Treatment

o Rigorous exclusion diets are required to give the gut a chance to heal. For all children with behavioural problems, food colourings, preservatives and flavour enhancers must be removed from the diet. In some cases, there is sensitivity to salicylates: see the Salicylates chart in Part 7. Wheat, yeast and dairy are also common sensitivities.

o The constitutional medicine is vital for these children. This, in combination with an exclusion diet, gives the best possible outcome. Often nosodes are needed. In the case of disturbed gut flora, the bowel nosodes can initiate a deep healing response. For further discussion of bowel nosodes see [127]. Common prescriptions for hyperactive or defiant behaviour in children are *Tuberculinum bov, Medorrhinum, Hyoscyamus and Tarentula*. Some of these are well described by Paul Herscu in *The Homeopathic Treatment of Children.*

o Another common problem is the prevalence of intestinal parasites: see *Abdominal Pain in Children* at [25]. This is the most common cause of night terrors in children (apart from identifiable reasons from the child's life story). Look for itchy nose or rectum, teeth grinding, unexplained abdominal pain,

persistent unformed stools, to confirm this diagnosis. Unexplained tantrums or irritability, with one or more of the above symptoms, should prompt one to suspect intestinal parasites.
o Children with a strong family history of multiple allergy or sensitivity often respond well to *Tuberculinum Bov 1M*. See the discussion of allergy vs sensitivity at [89] ff.
o Children with gut-brain disorders may have vaccinosis. See *Vaccinosis* at [33].
o A great many children with persistent diarrhoea respond positively to either the protocol for parasite elimination (see [25]) or treatment for the side effects of a childhood vaccination (see [33]). Still others require dietary modification: see the discussion on food sensitivity at [93] and [103].
o Probiotics are needed in many cases to restore the gut flora after generation exposure to antibiotics, as mentioned above. Bowel nosodes can make a large impact on gut flora quality and can be given in conjunction with the constitutional medicine and nutritional interventions.

Other factors which have a potential to affect behaviour:
o Emotional
o Teething
o Undetected ear infection
o Headache
o Hypoglycaemia
o Constipation
o Silent reflux
o Food sensitivities.

Summary of factors for treating children with gut-brain disorders:
o *Nutrition:* Check zinc status. Nutrients are not absorbed well if the patient has chronic diarrhoea.
o *Exclusion diet:* Wheat, dairy, yeast, food colourings and preservatives. In some cases, salicylates.
o *Intestinal parasites:* see [25].
o *Allergy:* Family history of allergy or food sensitivity.
o *Vaccinosis:* See [33].
o This material is expanded fully in Gamble, J *Mastering Homeopathy 2: The Treatment of Irritable Bowel Syndrome* (2006).

For a case example see Part 5, Case 1.

WHY BABIES CRY

See also Abdominal Pain in Children at [24]

[40]
Oesophageal Reflux
- *Aethusa cynapium 200:* Specific for reflux in babies, where the baby is not able to tolerate the mother's milk. This is the first remedy to use where babies are vomiting after feeding.
- *Bismuth 6:* If the vomiting occurs a long time after feeding and *Aethusa* has failed.
- If symptoms persist, suspect food sensitivity. Check for a family history of food sensitivity and eliminate that food from the mother's diet. The most common food sensitivities are wheat, dairy and yeast. Other sensitivities are peanut, egg, soy and salicylate. Whilst the mother's milk is the best food source for babies, if the child has a food sensitivity, that food must be withdrawn from the mother's diet.
- Silent reflux is particularly difficult to identify because no regurgitation is evident. The only reliable evidence may be that the baby cries after feeding.

If the child cries many hours after feeding, then colic is more likely to be the cause.

[41]
Colic
Flatulence, tympanic abdomen and pain.
- *Lycopodium 30 or 200*: Flatulence, plus aggravation late afternoon.
- *Colocynthis 200*: Where the baby is better from being placed over the parent's shoulder or lying on the stomach.
- *Morgan Pure 30:* In stubborn cases, where the child is unable to tolerate the breast milk, and there may be multiple food sensitivities, the bowel nosode *Morgan Pure 30* can cure.

See the comments at [38] ff in regard to food sensitivities.

[42]
Uretal reflux
There may be no symptoms at all, yet the crying will always stop once a course of antibiotics is given. This will lead the doctor to presume the problem was an ear infection. However evidence can only be found with analysis of the baby's urine. A surprising number of cases of persistent crying have turned out to be uretal reflux or cystitis. Most cases respond well to *Cantharis 200*. If *Cantharis* does not work, try *Medorrhinum 1M*. Since there is possibility of kidney damage in chronic uretal reflux referral for medical assessment is essential.

[43]
Ear infection & Teething

Look for ear tugging or brushing, which is a common sign in ear infection in babies. Take particular note if the DPT (or DTPa) vaccination has recently been given.

- *Pulsatilla 30:* In ear pain associated with a cold or mucus, without fever or inflammation.
- *Ferrum phos 200:* If low fever accompanies ear pain.
- *Belladonna 3 or 200:* If there is high fever. Always use *Belladonna 3* if the tympanum is red.
- *Chamomilla 30:* If associated with teething. If *Chamomilla* fails, use *Kreosotum 200.*
- *Gelsemium 200:* In a small number of cases where children cannot settle during teething, try *Gelsemium 200* (if low fever) or *Coffea 200* (if there is a history of easily starting from sleep).
- *Gelsemium 200:* In older children who become incontinent during teething. There may an accompanying fever.

HEADACHES IN CHILDREN

[44]
Overview
Children can have persistent headaches which are unresponsive to osteopathy and other methods of treatment. Careful case taking is necessary as there may be psychological or abuse issues which are being somaticised as headaches. They could also be sinus headaches: check for tenderness of the facial bones or the presence of blocked nose or mucus with the headache.

Intestinal parasites can also cause headaches. Check for rectal or nasal itch, teeth grinding, unexplained night terrors or abdominal pains. If all these avenues of enquiry fail, as indeed they may, the best remedy for unexplained persistent headaches in children is *Calcarea phos 200*, repeated regularly. If the child has difficulty sleeping, calcium phosphate can be given in a material dose at bedtime. Headaches and insomnia in children may point to *Carcinosin* if the symptoms agree.

[45]
Treatment
- *Calcarea phos 200*: The remedy *par excellence* for childhood headaches of unknown origin.
- *Carcinosin 200*: Headaches + insomnia.
- *Spigelia 200*: Headaches associated with intestinal parasites.
- *Sanguinaria 200*: Headaches associated with sinusitis, unless there are specific indications for another remedy.
- *Natrum carb 200:* Headache or sinus headache worse in the heat.
- *Natrum mur 200*: Headache starting in the morning and worsening as the day proceeds.
- *Melilotis 30c*: Headache with severe vomiting.

PART 2: ILLNESSES IN WOMEN

CANDIDA & VAGINITIS

[46]
GIT candidiasis
This is commonly found in women who suffer from vaginal candida (monilia).

Clinical presentation
Two or more symptoms of:
- Abdominal bloating
- Sugar craving and/or intolerance
- Mood swings
- History of thrush or vaginitis
- Fatigue.

[47]
Diagnosis
GIT candida symptoms are similar to hypoglycaemic symptoms. Where the patient has tiredness and dizziness or headache more than two hours after eating with a craving for sugar, think first of a disturbance in sugar metabolism, rather than candidiasis. If there is a history of vaginal candidiasis with leucorrhoea or itching, then think of GIT candida. Of course, both syndromes may occur concurrently.

[48]
Treatment
- *Candida albicans 20M*: Twice daily for 10 days.
- *Lycopodium 30:* If there is flatulence and abdominal bloating, also give *Lycopodium* three times daily.

Make sure the patient steadfastly avoids sugar, and eats a snack containing protein every two hours throughout the day. Fresh fruit is safe provided it is with a meal. It is not necessary to remove yeast from the diet unless the patient has a specific allergy or sensitivity to it.

One normally sees improvement after 10 days. If there is no improvement, it may be necessary to review the diagnosis, or consider a symptom specific remedy such as *Kreosotum* (for vaginal thrush).

Once the patient has improved on *Candida albicans 20M* give the following course for a further 10 days:
- Increase *Candida albicans* to 50M twice daily and reduce *Lycopodium 30* to twice daily or less frequent doses depending on symptoms.

This protocol may need to be repeated. In the meantime a sugar-free diet is required and attention to stress may be needed. Constitutional treatment will need to follow.

Other medicines often required:

- *Kreosotum 200*: For persistent vaginal itch.
- If *Kreosotum* fails, consider *Nitric ac 200*, which has prickly, itchy pains.
- *Arsenicum 200:* Where there is vaginal soreness and inflammation is more prominent than itching.

See Vaginitis below.

If there is persistent leucorrhoea with a white, yeasty discharge, it will usually improve on the *Candida nosode/Lycopodium* regime. If not, see Leucorrhoea at [52] for a specific prescription.

When the above regime is complete, lifestyle advice, especially with regard to stress, is needed. The diet should have refined sugars excluded and the patient should eat two-hourly snacks until the fatigue improves.

If flatulence persists, there may be hypochlorhydria (see Hypochlorhydria at [142]). Consider supplementing with digestive enzymes after food or gentian tincture before each meal: see [142].

[49]
Vaginal candidiasis & vaginitis

Clinical presentation
Vaginal itch with or without leucorrhoea; inflammation of labial and vaginal tissue. Diabetes, pregnancy and use of the oral contraceptive pill can predispose to vaginal candidiasis.

[50]
Diagnosis
It is necessary to differentiate simple vaginitis or leucorrhoea from sexually transmitted diseases (STDs). Diagnosis is confirmed by swab culture. See Leucorrhoea at [52]. Monilia candida should be differentiated from cystitis, which may cause only low grade discomfort, with dysuria: see [77].

[51]
Treatment

- *Kreosotum 200:* The main medicine: itch+++ often with a white, yeasty discharge.

Other medicines:

- *Arsenicum 200:* No itch, but vaginitis with inflammation and soreness of tissues, with minimal discharge.
- *Nitric ac 200*: Itch or pain which is 'prickly'. May have a ropy discharge.
- *Platina 6:* Where the vaginal wall is extremely sensitive to the slightest touch.

For other medicines see Leucorrhoea at [52].

LEUCORRHOEA

[52]
Clinical presentation
A persistent white, yellow or green vaginal discharge resulting from inflammation or congestion. See the chart below.

[53]
Differential diagnosis
The type of discharge helps to differentiate a leucorrhoea from other causes:

o A *yeasty white* discharge, especially associated with itching, is likely to be candida (monilia). See [46]. Other possibilities are cervical erosion and cervical polyps.
o A *watery* discharge is likely to be genital herpes.
o A *yellow* discharge is often a sign of bacterial infection, eg chlamydia. This may point to underlying inflammation, such as cervicitis, or pelvic inflammatory disease (PID). In vaginitis, the tissues appear red, sore, and possibly itchy. If there is pain and bleeding on intercourse, or persistent bloody discharge not associated with menses, it needs to be medically investigated to rule out malignancy. A non-malignant condition which produces this result is cervical erosion, which is more common in women taking synthetic hormones.
o A *yellow-green* discharge with foul odour may be gonorrhoea.
o A *thin, green or greyish-white foul* discharge which adheres to the vaginal walls may be gardnerella.
o A profuse, *green* vaginal discharge is likely to be trichomonas, which is a sexually transmitted disease. Trichomonas can also cause cystitis. The discharge is frequently bubbly or frothy and has a foul odour.

Causations of Vaginal Discharges other than Leucorrhoea

Discharge	Causation
Watery & thin	Atrophic vaginitis
	Genital herpes
White	Candida
Yellow & odourless	Chlamydia
Yellow-green & foul odour	Gonorrhoea
Green	Trichomonas
	Gardnerella
Bloody	Cancer

[54]
Treatment

- *Kreosotum 200:* The main remedy whenever itching accompanies the discharge.
- *Arsenicum 200:* If there is vaginitis without itching, but with soreness and inflammation.
- *Nitric ac 200:* Sharp, sticking or pinching pains, especially if at the muco-dermal junction.

Other remedies:
- *Alumina 200*: Very watery, acrid discharge, worse daytime. There is bearing down felt in the lower abdomen, rawness of the parts. The discharge may also be white, but not offensive.
- *Syphilinum 30:* The discharge is offensive and worse at night. The patient has a sickly appearance.
- *Sepia 200*: Watery or thick, lumpy discharge worse after urination. Usually associated with menstrual irregularities, eg dysmenorrhoea.
- *Borax 30*: Discharge which feels hot and itchy. Discharge is gelatinous, gummy and thick, like raw egg.

[55]
Summary

- *Kreosotum 200*: Main remedy; itch+++.
- *Arsenicum 200*: Vaginitis with soreness and inflammation.

OESTROGEN DOMINANCE

[56]
Clinical presentation
It is important to remember the prevalence of oestrogen dominance and the health problems its causes. Use of the oral contraceptive pill (OCP) and hormone replacement therapy (HRT) is widespread in the western world. We also have the presence of xeno-oestrogens from plastics and exposure to oestrogenic chemicals in the environment. It is therefore important to consider the presence of oestrogen dominance as an iatrogenic disease, just as with any other drug.

If a woman presents with anxiety, or facial eruptions which are aggravated mid cycle or during menses, look for other symptoms of oestrogen dominance to confirm the diagnosis.

The main symptoms are:
- o Premenstrual migraine
- o Menorrhagia
- o Metrorrhagia
- o Anxiety
- o Insomnia
- o Body ache
- o Low libido
- o Fatigue
- o Fibroids and endometrial growth
- o Weight gain
- o Foggy thinking.

[57]
Differential diagnosis
Other hormonal imbalances; hypothyroidism; anaemia; anxiety; non-hormone exacerbated emotional issues; GIT candidiasis; uterine and ovarian pathology.

[58]
Treatment
Where hypothyroidism is apparent, the case will often benefit from commencing with repeated doses of:
- *Thyroidinum 200.*

Discontinue the oral contraceptive pill or HRT. The effect of these synthetic chemicals can be quickly and easily removed with:
- *Folliculinum 30*: Once daily for one to two weeks. *Folliculinum* is specific for removing synthetic oestrogens.

Folliculinum has aggravation of symptoms premenstrually or at mid-cycle, which can include:
- Facial eruptions (including unexplained flushing in young women)
- Flatulence
- Mood swings
- Palpitation
- Anxiety
- Period pain
- Breast engorgement
- Weight gain.

Folliculinum is often aggravated from heat. It is not recommended in low potencies (below 6c) in oestrogen dominance, as these may stimulate the release of oestrogen.

If the oestrogen dominance is present but it is not iatrogenic, the preferred remedy is:
- *Cimicifuga 30*: Give regularly for one or two months. If the symptoms are severe, use *Cimicifuga 200*. *Cimicifuga* keynotes are: agitation, restlessness and crampy or electric-type pain. Aggravation is experienced during the menses.

After the oestrogen dominance is corrected, a second prescription is usually needed, based on the individual symptoms remaining.
- *Sepia 200:* The main remedy for dysmenorrhoea and menorrhagia. *Sepia* is effective if facial eruptions persist which are aggravated at menses. For more discussion on dysmenorrhoea and menorrhagia: see [64].

If anxiety persists, higher potencies of *Folliculinum or Cimicifuga* can be tried. If these fail, the patient needs a constitutional prescription.

There are many other treatment options for female hormonal imbalances. The work of Kathy Harris is a good resource for these. (See Bibliography.)

[59]
Summary
- *Folliculinum 30*: Iatrogenic oestrogen dominance.
- *Cimicifuga 30*: Non-iatrogenic oestrogen dominance.

Follow with:
- *Sepia 200*: Facial eruptions aggravated at menses, dysmenorrhoea and menorrhagia.

MASTITIS

[60]
Clinical presentation
Localised pain, inflammation and swelling of the breast due to obstruction of the milk ducts, often with fever and occasionally a purulent nipple discharge. There are tender nodules and erythema. The may be high fever and chills. Mastitis can have a sudden onset with mild to very severe pain. Mastitis usually occurs during breastfeeding.

[61]
Differential diagnosis
See Breast Lumps at [67].

[62]
Treatment
Breast-feeding women should continue to express their milk.
- *Bryonia 30:* The main remedy where there is severe tenderness or pain.
- *Belladonna 30:* If there is also a fever or any sign of inflammation (with local redness). Streaks may radiate from the nipple.
- *Hepar sulph 200:* In cases where there is a purulent nipple discharge, coupled with extreme contact sensitivity.
- *Phytolacca 200:* If the pain radiates to the axilla, or if there are multiple firm lumps associated with the mastitis.

[63]
Summary
- *Bryonia 30:* The main remedy for pain.
- *Belladonna 30*: Pain with inflammation or fever.
- *Hepar sulph 200*: Contact hypersensitivity with purulence.
- *Phytolacca 200*: Pain radiates, or there are multiple firm lumps.

DYSMENORRHOEA & MENORRHAGIA

[64]
Clinical presentation
Dysmenorrhoea: menstrual pain. Menorrhagia: heavy and/or prolonged bleeding.

[65]
Differential diagnosis
Endometriosis & adenomyosis; uterine pathology (eg polyp, fibroid etc); pelvic inflammatory disease; pregnancy; missed miscarriage.

[66]
Treatment
- *Sepia 200*: Where no other remedies are clear, start with *Sepia,* repeated twice per week, for at least two months, but not taken during the menses. It reduces both period pain and heavy flow. The presence of 'bearing down' sensation described in the materia medicas is not required to prescribe *Sepia.* We have prescribed *Sepia* more often than other remedies in the absence of other individualising symptoms.
- *Lilium tig 200*: Menses are heavy, with bearing down pains (*Sep*). There are often large clots. Bleeding stops when the patient is still (= aggravation from motion) (*Croc, Erig, Helon. Sab).* A concomitant symptom is urgent desire for stool.
- *Sabina 200*: Period pain extends to or from the sacrum to the uterus. This remedy is useful where there is a history of infection, such as after a termination of pregnancy. In severe cases, there is bleeding from any movement (*Lil-t*) or from sexual excitement. Menstrual flow may be in paroxysms, and there may be severe headache with the period. This remedy can be considered where there is a history of repeated abortions, or a history of infection, eg pelvic inflammatory disease.
- *Staphysagria 200*: The period pain or heavy bleeding has commenced after a tubal ligation. In these cases, always start with *Staphysagria 200* or higher, which is specific for the after-effects of surgery. Give repeated doses for several weeks.
- *Folliculinum 30*: When symptoms commence after starting the contraceptive pill, the pill should be discontinued and *Folliculinum 30* given for several weeks.
- *Secale 200*: Secale affords great relief where one period lasts almost to the next one, giving the patient only a week or so in the month without bleeding. Pain is often a minimal symptom.
- *Helonias 200*: There is clear atony or engorgement of the uterus, with prostration and weakness, possibly anaemia, following childbirth, abortion or miscarriage. The patient is aware of her uterus with every movement. The pelvic floor feels heavy, sore and the menstrual blood is dark and offensive.

- *Caulophyllum 200*: As with *Helonias*, there is engorgement or hypertrophy of the uterus, which may follow childbirth or multiple childbirths. However, it is not a fibroid remedy and will thus benefit younger women. There may be subinvolution of the uterus, which produces ongoing discomfort in the pelvic floor and pain radiating into the legs.
- *Thlaspi Bursa Pastoralis*: The first remedy to consider in menopausal women with fibroids, heavy bleeding and large clots. There may be uterine pain when rising. It is best taken in tincture or the lower potencies, up to 30C.
- *Pulsatilla 30 or 200*: Consider this remedy when there is a strong history of amenorrhoea or irregularity of the menses.
- *Cimicifuga 30*: Pain increases as the flow increases. Large clots.

For inter-cycle bleeding:
- *Bovista 200:* Polymenorrhagia or metrorrhagia.
- *Trillium:* Polymenorrhagia.
- *Sabina 200:* Metrorrhagia after the least movement (compare *Lilium-t).*

Summary
- *Sepia 200:* The main remedy.
- *Lilium tig 200:* Aggravation from movement.
- *Sabina 200:* Pain between sacrum and uterus. History of infection.
- *Staphisagria 200:* After surgery.
- *Folliculinum 30:* Side effects from synthetic oestrogen.
- *Secale 200:* Protracted bleeding for most of the month.
- *Helonias 200:* Uterine engorgement with awareness of the womb.
- *Caulophylum 200:* Uterine engorgement in younger women.
- *Thlaspi Bursa Pastoralis MT to 30:* Fibroids especially at menopause.
- *Pulsatilla 30:* History of amenorrhoea or irregularity.
- *Cimicifuga 30:* Pain increases with the flow.
- *Bovista, Trillium & Sabina:* Inter-cycle bleeding.

BREAST LUMPS

[67]
Differential diagnosis
o *Fibrocystic breast disease*: This is the most common cause of breast lumps. The nodule is smooth, mobile, firm and increases in dimensions with the menstrual cycle. Symptoms may also occur premenstrually, and in some cases there is a clear nipple discharge
o *Breast cancer*: Malignant nodules are usually hard, fixed to the underlying tissue (ie non-mobile), with nipple retraction and dimpling as a consequence. A nipple discharge may be bloody. Lumps such as these should always be referred for biopsy.
o *Breast abcess*: A localised, inflamed, hot, exquisitely painful lump often with raised systemic temperature and malaise.
o *Mastitis*: The breast feels warm (not hot), with tender nodules, swelling and erythema. There may be fever and chills.
o *Fibroadenoma*: Also called a 'breast mouse' because it is slippery when palpated (unlike breast cancer which is not). The nodule is usually single, round, elastic, with well defined edges. It is usually painless.

Treatment

[68]
Fibrocystic breast disease
• *Sepia 200 alternating with Conium 3* on alternate days particularly when there are accompanying menstrual symptoms such as dysmenorrhoea. If Conium 3 only gives a partial improvement, one should increase the potency to 200c and give that once every 2nd day for at least one month, either in alternation with Sepia or alone.
• *Phytolacca 200:* If local pain is the dominant symptom.

[69]
Breast cancer
Any lump which is hard, has irregular edges and does not move freely when palpated should be referred for medical investigation.

[70]
Breast abcess
• *Hepar sulph 200:* The main remedy, especially where there is exquisite pain.
• *Belladonna 3:* If redness and fever are dominant.

These two remedies can be alternated with good effect.

[71]
Mastitis is discussed at [60].

[72]
Fibroadenoma
- *Conium 3*: Works well where the nodule is hard. Alternate with *Sepia 200* as described above if there are concomitant menstrual symptoms.
- *Mercurius viv 200*: For a large cystic mass.
- *Phytolacca 200*: For a multi-nodular mass, even where there is no pain.

All the above pathologies may take a long time to disperse with remedies. Repeat the remedies regularly as described in the 'How to Use' section.

MORNING SICKNESS

[75]
Differential diagnosis
Gallbladder stasis; food poisoning; influenza; allopathic medication; travel sickness.

[76]
Treatment
- *Colchicum 30*: Nausea at the smell, or mere thought, of food.
- *Phosphorus 200*: Vomiting+++.
- *Tabacum 200*: Constant nausea without vomiting. Dizziness, pallor, coldness and intermittent sweats.
- *Cocculus 200:* Nausea resulting from lack of sleep.
- *Symphoricarpus 200*: Vomiting +++ and aggravation from motion.
- *Medorrhinum 200:* Obstinate or unresponsive cases.

CYSTITIS

[77]
Clinical presentation
Dysuria: pain is normally experienced during urination which is often described as burning or 'peeing razor blades'; frequency and urging. In severe cases there is visible haematuria. Fever may also be present.

[78]
Differential diagnosis
Urethritis; nephritis; uterine prolapse; pelvic abcess; malignancy;dysmenorrhoea.

[79]
Treatment
- *Cantharis 200*: Specific for cystitis and covers the vast majority of cases. This remedy can be repeated for months if there is chronic recurring cystitis. May also be used in children.
- *Medorrhinum 200 or 1M:* Chronic cystitis particularly if there is a history of sexually transmitted disease. Also for children with history of severe nappy rash.
- *Benzoic ac 200:* Occasionally needed where the urine has a pungent smell which remains after the toilet is flushed.
- *Sarsaparilla 30:* For pain at the close of urination.

PART 3: GENERAL ILLNESSES

ASTHMA

[80]
Overview &
Clinical presentation

This chapter applies to asthma in children and adults, except where stated. Asthma is now commonly referred to as a disease of affluence, as the incidence of asthma is greater in developed countries. Asthma can improve when dietary factors are addressed. For example, reduction in dairy foods, wheat and increasing whole grain foods and good quality omega-3 oils often lead to a good overall improvement. Refer to the dietary appendices in Part 7.

Asthma may be divided into two categories:
o *Extrinsic asthma* refers to asthma triggered by an allergy.
o *Intrinsic asthma* has no external triggers.

The majority of asthma patients suffer from extrinsic asthma. While it may not always be possible to identify any or all of the triggers, some common ones are food additives eg MSG; airborne allergens eg mould spores, pollens and dust and some foods such as strawberries, yeast and crustaceans.

Allergic patients may also have atopic eczema, hay fever and migraine. The precise allergens need to be identified. Where a small number of food allergens are identified, they can be excluded from the diet whilst those same allergens are given homeopathically: see the desensitising section for Sinusitis at [104]. Even when desensitisation has been successful, constitutional treatment is needed to completely resolve the allergic diathesis. Otherwise the patient will next develop allergy to a different allergen and one has to repeat the treatment. See the detailed discussion of allergy at [89] ff.

General measures to reduce allergy:
o *Omega-3 polyunsaturated fatty acids:* such as flax (linseed) oil and deep sea fish, help reduce inflammation.
o *Bowel, liver health:* See [38] for a discussion of the importance of functional intestinal function and immunity. Liver health ensures correct removal of lymph.
o *Reduce excess mucus*: This may include avoidance of dairy foods.
o *Reduce emotional stress*: Most asthmatics experience aggravation of symptoms during times of stress. Stress induces the production of proinflammatory cytokines and thus chronic stress results in reduced resistance to allergies and infection.

Clinical presentation
There is an episodic (expiratory) wheeze and dyspnoea due to temporary airway obstruction and possibly inflammation. In mild cases there is a persistent, short dry cough with no obvious wheeze, especially in children. Many asthmatics are worse with changes in weather, cold weather and, if extrinsic, worse in spring. Most patients with intrinsic asthma are worse after exercise. A post-viral wheeze is not asthma without further evidence of asthmatic symptoms.

[81]
Differential diagnosis

Children *(see table below for symptom differentials)*
o Pneumonia
o Croup
o Epiglottitis
o Whooping cough
o Bronchitis & bronchiolitis.

Adults *(see table below for symptoms differentials)*
o Bronchitis
o Pneumonia
o Bronchiectasis
o Pleurisy
o Congestive heart failure.

Other symptom differentials
o No lung sounds during an asthma attack (neoplasm or effusion)
o Localised wheeze (congenital abnormality or foreign body)
o Relationship with feeding in a child (gastro-oesophageal reflux)
o Dyspnoea unresponsive to treatment: consider suppurative lung diseases: eg bronchiectasis, cystic fibrosis
o Emphysema.

Less common causes of dyspnoea
o Multiple pulmonary emboli
o Hypersensitivity neumonitis
o Allergic bronchopulmonary aspergillosis
o Tuberculosis
o Pulmonary sarcoidosis.

See the table of symptom differentials on the next page.

Table of Symptom Differentials

Illness	Fever	Age group	Auscult	Percuss	Appear	Cough	Dysp-noea	Other
Broncho-pneu-monia (upper)	•Yes •No chill •No rigor	•Childre n	•Diffuse bilateral rhonchi	•Normal both sides	•Flapping nostrils. •Tissue Retrac-tion.	•Yes, pain-less	•Yes •Rapid breathin g	•No chest pain. •Grunting expiration . •Fast pulse
Lobar-Pneu-monia (lower)	•Yes •Chill •Rigor	•Adults (occ child)	•Crepitus one side •Friction rub poss-ible	•Dull affected side	•Mouth breathing •Chest restricted one side	•Yes, pain-ful	•Yes	•Grunting expiration •Fast pulse
Bronchial Asthma	•No	•All ages	•Wheeze •Rhonchi	•Normal	•Cyanosi s if severe	•Some-times	•Yes	•Short in-breath-long out
Bronchio-litis	•Some-times	•Childre n	•Rhonchi •Crepitus	•Normal	•Normal	•Some-times	•No •Rapid breathin g	•Long expiration
Congest-ive heart failure	•No	•Usually adults	•Basal crepitus	•Normal	•Pitting oedema of legs. •Cyanosi s	•No	•Yes	•Liver tender & palpable
Pleurisy	•No	•Usually adults	•Pleural rub	•Normal		•Minimal	•No	•Pain only symptom
Croup	•Not commo n	•Childre n	•Inspiratio n stridor	•Normal	•Supra-sternal retraction	•Barking	•Yes	•Hypoxic if severe
Epiglotti-tis*	•Not commo n	•Childre n	•Insp/exp snoring stridor	•Normal	•Sits up •Open mouth	•No	•Yes	•Hypoxic •Won't swallow
Whoop-ing Cough	•Initial stage only	•Childre n	•Fine crepitus		•Red face •Cyanosi s in infants	•Whoop sound on in-breath •Parox-ysmal		•Apnoea in infants

© Jon Gamble 2004

*hospitalisation required; do not use tongue depressors

[82]
Treatment: Acute

When patients seek homeopathic treatment for asthma they may already be taking corticosteroids as 'preventers' and bronchodilators for managing acute bronchospasm. Alternatively, they may be taking a leukotriene antagonist such as *Singulair. Patients should keep taking their allopathic medication whilst taking the homeopathic medicine.* The latter must be repeated regularly at the commencement of treatment, at least until improvement is established. In these cases, we give the patient a mixture comprising:

• *Bryonia 30 and Arsenicum 3 combined* ('asthma mix'): Use in place of bronchodilators. Patients are asked to use their bronchodilator if needed, but are encouraged to take this mix before doing so. In this way, the psychological and physiological dependence on the bronchodilator is lessened slowly without causing distress to the patient. Initially the above mix may have little effect but with repeated use its effect is gradually felt, and reliance on bronchodilators is reduced.

Never withdraw a patient's corticosteroid medication when commencing homeopathic treatment. It can only be withdrawn very slowly once clear improvement is seen. The effect of the homeopathic remedy will not be diminished by the allopathic medication provided the homeopathics are repeated regularly.

[83]
Treatment: Chronic

- *Tuberculinum bov 1M:* Where there is a clear allergic diathesis to *multiple* airborne or contact allergens, *Tuberculinum bov* can be repeated periodically. In highly allergic patients, the first dose can cause an aggravation of symptoms: warn the patient in advance! Start with 1M potency and continue with that potency once weekly while it is of benefit, then increase up the usual scale. *Tuberculinum bov* is especially indicated where there is an allergy to animal fur, and of course can be considered if there are other indicators for the tubercular miasm.
- *Bacillinum:* If the patient is excessively hot: use *Bacillinum* instead of *Tuberculinum.*
- *Kali carb 200:* If *Tuberculinum* is not indicated or does not act, and there are no other individualising symptoms, begin treatment with *Kali carb*, repeated every second day, and reducing frequency only upon improvement. Patients may have had symptoms which are long since suppressed or forgotten, owing to the length of time they have been using allopathic medication. It can be very difficult to discern individualising symptoms and arrive at a confident prescription in these cases. *Kali carb* has many of the classic asthma symptoms, including aggravation from cold weather and atmospheric changes. While *Kali carb* will not cure every asthma case, it goes a long way in improving the patient's overall condition whilst permitting reduction of their allopathic medication. Old symptoms may re-emerge with the slow reduction in allopathic medication. It is then easier to discern the constitutional medicine (if other than *Kali carb*). In any case, while *Kali carb* is effective in reducing the incidence of asthma attacks, it should be continually repeated at increasingly greater intervals, and in the same potency.
- *Psorinum 1M*: Where asthma and eczema alternate, the psoric miasm may be causative, in which case *Psorinum* can be used intercurrently, both to stimulate immunity and decrease reactivity.
- *Ammonium carb 200*: The focus of the disease rests in the sinuses, with chronic blocked nose and wheezing, sneezing and nightly aggravation.
- *Causticum 200*: Marked aggravation from winds in empathic patients.
- *Arsenicum 3 or 6*: Strongly allergic asthma with related symptoms such as contact dermatitis, itchy eyes and sneezing *without* a blocked nose. If there are '*Arsenicum*' generals, the 200th potency may be more effective.

- *Natrum sulph 30 or 200*: 'Sycotic' asthma with clear aggravation from damp weather. (Compare *Medhorrhinum.*)
- *Bowel nosodes:* The bowel nosodes *Mutabile* and *Morgan (Bach)* are also indicated. *Mutabile* is specific for alternation of symptoms, such as asthma and eczema. The keynote for *Morgan (Bach)* is asthma and eczema.
- *Aspidosperma 3x:* While not specifically an asthma remedy, this affords symptomatic relief for dyspnoea caused by **emphysema**.

[87]
Children
The above remedies can also be prescribed for children. For asthma in children, always investigate vaccinosis as a likely cause. Vaccine-induced asthma responds to the protocol described at [34].

The same asthma mix (*Bryonia 30 & Arsenicum 3 mixed*) can be used for children, but in young children whose asthma is associated with a loose, phlegmy chest (rattling cough), *Ipecac 30* is more effective. Common children's remedies are described below.

Mouth breathing in children may be a precursor to the development of asthma. Children must be encouraged to breathe properly and their mouths may have to be taped with micropore tape for specified periods in the day to encourage this. If the child cannot breathe through the nose, they probably have adenoid hypertrophy:

- *Baryta carb 200:* Inability to nose-breathe due to enlarged adenoids. If nasal examination reveals nasal polyps: see [97].
- *Calcarea carb 30:* Frequent colds plus adenoid hypertrophy. Repeat once daily until improvement, then reduce the frequency to every second day.

Other remedies often used in children's asthma:
- *Phosphorus 30 or 200*: In frightened, anxious children who aggravate from cold or changes in weather.
- *Silicea 200*: For children who are chronically sick with ear, nose and throat (ENT) diseases, with chronically enlarged tonsils and adenoids. The '*Silicea*' child may be fine-boned.
- *Ipecac 30*: As mentioned above, use *Ipecac* for asthma in young children who have a loose, phlegmy chest cough or rattly rhonchi.
- *Medorrhinum 30 or 200*: 'hyperactive' children, never still, who may also be aggressive.

Medicine may need to be repeated for months. Many of these children will benefit from a dairy-free diet (look for lymphatic rosary in the iris), while a smaller number will benefit from a wheat-free diet.

[88]
Summary

- *Kali carb 200*: The main remedy for **adult** asthma.
- *Tuberculinum bov 1M*: Allergic diathesis.
- *Ammonium carb 200*: Sinus symptoms with blocked nose and wheezing worse at night.
- *Causticum 200*: Aggravation from winds in empathic patients.
- *Bryonia 30 + Arsenicum 3* (mixed) ('asthma mix'): For acute wheeze and cough. To be used as needed to reduce reliance on Ventolin for **children or adults.**
- *Natrum sulph 30/200:* Sycotic asthma.
- *Calcarea carb 30 or Phosphorus 30 or 200*: The main remedies for **childhood** asthma.
- *Ipecac 30:* Asthma in **children** who have loose, rattly chests (not dry rhonchi).

ALLERGY

[89]
Overview
Patients who have had poor results managing chronic allergies (atopic conditions) or where 'allergies' have been incorrectly diagnosed, often turn to homeopathy as a last resort.

Atopic illnesses, which include the asthma/eczema/hay fever triad, are characterised by a pronounced reaction or sensitivity to specific environmental triggers. *Allergic* reactions occur wherever there is a *histamine* reaction.

Some cases of 'allergy' stem from disordered gut function, so treatment of the GIT may be necessary. Consider the treatment discussions for Irritable Bowel Syndrome at [148]; Behavioural Problems in Children at [38] and see the discussion of the Bowel Nosodes at [127].

Genetic factors (miasmatic tendencies)
The causes of atopy are not fully understood. A parental history of allergy may contribute to a generalised risk for their children. Maternal atopy is more strongly related to the children's asthma and hay fever than paternal atopy. Taking a detailed case history will determine the patient's familial and childhood history which is a useful tool in evaluating a predisposition to atopy.

Why is allergy so prevalent?
Exposure to animals in childhood reduces the likelihood of atopy developing. Exposure to normal childhood diseases also reduces the likelihood of atopy because exposure to these influences favours the production of the T helper cells Th1 (as opposed to Th2).

Repeated bacterial and viral infections during childhood protect against the development of allergic disease by enhancing Th1 development. Th1 cells favour IgA and IgG host immune responses which do not result in histamine reactions. But Th2 cells favour *IgE* host responses, which are directly involved in histamine responses. Th2 cell development is favoured when children are not exposed to the above factors.

Therefore, a child exposed to animals and the normal childhood diseases is less likely to develop histamine (or allergic) reactions than a child who is not exposed to these factors. Preventing such infections (eg via vaccination and antibiotics) *may increase the incidence of allergy*. Encourage parents to keep a pet in the house!

Allergy Tests
- *Skin prick test* – The most widely used method for testing a broad range of allergies. An intra-cutaneous method of testing commonly used to test for type I immediate hypersensitivity reaction to antigens.
- *Radioallergosorbent test (RAST)*: Used when direct skin testing is not possible due to skin irritation or disease. This test involves a known allergen to be mixed with a sample of the patient's serum. Any IgE specific allergen in

the serum will attach to the conjugate. The amount of radioactivity taken up by the conjugate will determine the level of IgE.

o *Patch tests*: A method used to test type IV delayed hypersensitivity reactions. Common allergens are applied under aluminum discs for two days and four days to the skin on the back. The skin is examined at two and four day intervals for any evidence of an eczematous reaction. If present, the result is indicative of type IV hypersensitivity to the allergen being tested. Patch tests are used for defining contact sensitivities (especially dust mite in eczema).

o *Serum IgE estimations*: This test has limited value because a patient may have a positive skin prick or RAST test and yet have normal IgE levels. Serum IgE is helpful in detecting chronic infection, as elevated IgE may suggest parasitic infestation or contact sensitivity.

Non-TGA approved allergy test devices:
o Acu-dermal testing devices (Vega, Listen, Q4, Afdat) etc.

Other:
o Applied kinesiology (muscle testing).

[90]
Differential diagnosis
Patients believe they have 'food allergies', or are told they have allergies, yet in our experience, most do not. What these people have are food sensitivities, which clear up when their gastro-intestinal problems are corrected. See Hypochlorhydria at [142]; Gastritis, Peptic ulcer and Indigestion at [135]; Biliary stasis at [144]; Irritable Bowel Syndrome at [148] and Intestinal Parasites at [25].

[91]
Iatrogenic Factors
Vaccination and antibiotics prevent natural host immune responses to childhood diseases. This may promote allergies, as described above. Early onset atopy increases the possibility of developing asthma.

[92]
Common allergens *(ie those which elicit a histamine or IgE response):*
o Mould
o Animal Fur
o Pollens
o Sulphites (Food Additives 221-3)
o Yeast
o MSG (Food Additive 621)
o Benzoate (Food Additive 210-13)
o Peanuts
o Strawberries (or other salicylates)
o Crustaceans.

[93]
Common chemical sensitivities *(not allergies: there is no histamine or IgE response):*
o Pesticides
o Petrochemicals
o Perfumes
o Cleaning Agents
o Paint
o Cigarette Smoke.

[94]
Food sensitivities *(not causing IgE response):*
o Yeast
o Wheat
o Cow's milk
o Strawberries (or other salicylates)
o Crustaceans.
Remember that a food intolerance or sensitivity is not an allergy: it does not produce histamine reactions.

[95]
Intestinal Parasites
Many patients with 'allergies' have eosinophilia showing in their blood tests. Eosinophilia may point to allergies, but it can also indicate intestinal parasites. Bowel disturbance such as flatulence, shifting abdominal pain, or other symptoms of irritable bowel syndrome, as well as 'allergies' which involve itching, hives or hay fever, may indicate the presence of intestinal parasites which, when removed, will remove the so-called allergies. This is far more common than is supposed.

[96]
Treatment

Airborne & Contact Allergies
After food allergens, airborne or contact substances are the next most common type of allergy.
• *Tuberculinum bov 1M:* Patients with multiple allergies require constitutional prescribing. In many patients, *Tuberculinum bov 1M* is a good place to begin when there are multiple allergies with a keynote of allergy to animal fur.
• *Histaminum plus allergen:* As described on the following page, the allergy desensitising protocol can be used for desensitising a patient to a specific allergen which causes a clear histamine reaction.
• *Bowel nosodes:* Consider a bowel nosode in the presence of allergies plus bowel symptoms instead of or after the allergy desensitising protocol. We have frequently, but not exclusively, used *Gaertner 30.*

- *Carcinosin 30/200:* Family history of cancer or diabetes; insomnia and fastidiousness. (Refer to Foubister's work in the Bibliography.)
- *Exclude where possible* the allergens from the patient's environment or diet whilst the treatment is being given. Challenge with one of the allergens once the treatment is concluded.

Allergy to a specific trigger can be corrected with the protocol described on the following page.

Intestinal parasites
- See the other treatment options at [25].
- If the patient with bowel symptoms plus allergies does not respond to the above regime, we would next recommend one of the bowel nosodes such as *Gaertner 30.*

Allergy Desensitising Protocol

Day	Medicine
1 3 5	Histaminum 10M
2 4 6	Allergen 200
7 9 11	Histaminum 50M
8 10 12	Allergen 30
13 15 17	Histaminum CM
14 16 18	Allergen 6

NB: the patient may develop 'allergy' type symptoms such as sneezing or hives early in this protocol. This is a positive sign that the protocol is working and need not be regarded as a true allergic reaction. This reaction normally passes without intervention within 24 hours.

The patient is theoretically no longer reactive to the allergen once this protocol is completed, although this procedure may have to be repeated in time if the allergic sensitivity returns.

If there is a history of anaphylaxis to the allergen, any challenge with the allergen after completion of this protocol should only be performed under medical supervision with appropriate emergency safeguards ready.

NASAL POLYPS

[97]
Clinical presentation
Most patients will happily avoid a surgical procedure for nasal polyps if given the option. As with all physical pathologies, remedies need to be repeated often to generate a cure of polyps. Frontal nasal polyps are more easily visible: always inspect the nasal passages when assessing blocked nose. Nasal blockage not caused by polyps needs a different remedy from that caused by polyps.

[98]
Differential diagnosis
Other causes of nasal obstruction: adenoid hypertrophy; sinusitis and rhinitis; foreign body; septal deviation; ozaena.

[99]
Treatment
The correct remedy can produce rapid results. In one case the patient's chronic polyps appeared on his tissue when blowing his nose, within three weeks of commencing treatment. The modalities and causations are important in choosing the correct remedy.

- *Ammonium carb 200*: Where there is clear nasal obstruction aggravated at night, sometimes with sneezing and/or asthma.
- *Teucrium 200*: There are no particular symptoms or modalities, other than specificity for nasal polyps. There may be post –nasal catarrh with obstruction. In other cases there may be a history of 'failure to thrive' or intestinal worms in children.
- *Kali bich 30:* The polyps have relapsed since surgical removal.
- *Staphysagria 200*: The polyps have formed for the *first time* since surgery (eg following a deviated septal correction). Give *Staphysagria* before using any of the other remedies, since it is specific for ailments originating from surgery.
- *Formica rufa 30*: Large polyps which visibly protrude.

SINUSITIS & RHINITIS

[100]
Clinical presentation
o *Sinusitis* has blocked nose with frontal headache, and there may be yellow or green *catarrh*.
o *Rhinitis* has watery *coryza*; frontal pain; sneezing; may have blocked nose; itching in nose, mouth or ears.
o *Catarrh* refers to a thick or purulent mucous discharge.
o *Coryza* refers to a watery discharge which is either bland or acrid.

[101]
Treatment: Acute
If there is no single, clear remedy for acute attacks, it is useful to mix together acute remedies for rhinitis so that the patient benefits from homeopathic remedies when s/he experiences an acute episode. In this way, the patient learns to rely on the homeopathics, with less allopathic medication to obstruct symptom presentation. This is similar to our treatment approach to asthma. *We have found that using acute homeopathic prescribing as needed does not have a deleterious effect on long-term homeopathic treatment.* If an acute remedy works well in addressing flare ups, there is no reason why one should not use that remedy as the chronic treatment, repeating it often for months with diminishing frequency as improvement sets in. An acute remedy will at least give the patient relief, and the practitioner time to find an effective deeper acting remedy.

  Always look for a seasonal or allergic factor in the presenting symptoms, since homeopathy works well in desensitising patients to either airborne or ingested allergens. The procedure for desensitising is described at [104], or if allergy is severe, use the protocol descried at [96].

• *Histaminum.* Use when there is a clear allergic response with sneezing, itching, acute inflammation and coryza. Use it in very high potency, 50M or higher. See the Allergy Desensitisation Protocol using *Histaminum* at [96].

  The table on the following page summarises the main acute remedies for sinusitis and rhinitis.

Acute Sinusitis and Rhinitis
Acute Treatment Summary

Rx	Nose	Sneeze	Itching	Coryza (watery)	Catarrh (thick)	Eyes	Chest
All-c 30	Not blocked	++	Eyes	Acrid, copious		Bland discharge	
Am-c 200	Blocked < night Polyps poss.	++		Bland			Wheeze
Ars-alb 6	Not blocked	++	Eyes, nose	Bland		Watery	Wheeze
Arum-t 30	Blocked; Pain @ root			Acrid, excoriat-ing. Bloody			
Arund 30	Anosmia	++	Roof of mouth. Nose			Itching	
Euphr 200				Bland, profuse		Acrid watery, red, profuse	
Kali-b 30	Pain root of nose; Anosmia; Blocked	+++		Watery & profuse	Post nasal, viscid green-yellow, fetid	Stringy discharge	
Nat-m 30	Blocked; Anosmia	+++		Violent, pro-longed			
Nux-v 30	Blocked <night, warm room; runs in daytime			Acrid	Catarrhal scraping in throat		Wheeze < eating; chest & head pain
Puls 30	Blocked <PM; fluent AM; pain @ root; Anosmia			Yes	Yellow, abundant Fetid	Thick, bland discharge	Dry cough in bed
Sabad 30	Sensitive to fragrances	++++		Bland; copious (tap!)		Redness; tears	
Wyeth 30			Posterior Nares				Dry cough burning & hacking

©Jon Gamble 2004

[102]
Treatment: Chronic

This section includes the following sub-categories:
- *[103] Food sensitivities*
- *[104] Airborne allergens*
- *[105] Bacterial infection*
- *[106] Drug miasms*
- *[107] Summary: chronic sinusitis with thick yellow or green mucus*
- *[108] Summary: chronic rhinitis with thin mucus*

Main Remedies:
- *Kali carb 200*: History of asthma or bronchitis. This chronic and deep-acting remedy can also be used for an acute flare-up in a person prone to chronic obstructive pulmonary disease or asthma. Frequent colds in adults, which result in asthma.
- *Sanguinaria 200:* The focus is the sinus headache. Heaviness, headache frontal, offensive yellow or green discharge, thick hawking, ozaena.
- *Pyrogenium 200*: Chronic sinusitis where a purulent nasal discharge is the focus.
- *Tuberculinum bov 1M:* Where there is multiple allergic sensitivity, and a strong family history of allergy or lung disease. (*Bacillinum* is preferable in hot patients).
- *Hepar sulph 200:* Sinus associated with swollen lymphatic glands, sore throat and cold air sensitivity.
- *Ammonium carb 200*: Sinus with blocked nose and sneezing, sometimes asthma, *with night aggravation.*
- *Pulsatilla 30 or 200*: Symptoms as described in the above table plus blockage of the middle ear.
- *Mercurius sol 200:* Green or yellow mucus with deep frontal pain and nasal crusts, nose blocked, swollen glands. Congestion is worse at night and better in the open air. Sometimes there is ear ache also worse at night.
- *Lycopodium 30:* Blocked nose worse at night with thick elastic plugs (*Kali-b).* Also for children with thick mucus and blocked nose.
- *Gelsemium 200:* Heavy feeling in sinuses, with sensation of dizziness, dull head and drooping eyelids.

When indicated remedies fail to act:
- *Nosodes:* If there is a purulent mucous discharge consider: *Sinusitis nosode, Streptococcinum & Staphylococcinum 10M* mixed in ascending potencies, standing alone or as an intercurrent remedy.
- *Psorinum 1M:* Try this remedy as an intercurrent when the indicated remedy is not working.
- *Morgan Pure/Bach 30*: Where there is bowel disturbance and/or asthma/eczema.

[103]
Chronic Treatment:

Food sensitivities

Allergy or sensitivity testing may reveal one or more food allergies. Often just one food sensitivity causes sinus symptoms. The most frequently implicated foods are: cow's milk products, yeast and wheat. *Simple removal is the first line of treatment.* Then consider constitutional treatment or specific allergen desensitisation. See the discussion of allergy at [89].

If food sensitivity (as opposed to allergy) is causing the sinus problem, it is necessary to improve gut function in order to cure the sinuses. See the discussions on Hypochlorhydria at [142], and Gallbladder Stasis at [144].

Where disordered bowel function is a feature, a bowel nosode often proves useful in opening the case.

Always check for zinc deficiency (white spots on fingernails) as well as nutritional implications, in the presence of food sensitivities or allergies.

[104]
Chronic Treatment:

Airborne allergens

Allergy testing may reveal one or more airborne allergies. Seasonal sinus problems suggest airborne allergens. Specific allergen desensitising is often useful.

If there are multiple allergies, with a family history of allergy and/or asthma, or where there is sensitivity to animal furs, *Tuberculinum bov 1M* is often curative. Be sure to warn the patient that this medicine can cause an initial sinus aggravation.

If there are only one or two specific allergens with clear coryza, sneezing or itching, another treatment plan is to use *Histaminum 50M* or CM.

The preferred method for allergy desensitisation is described at [96].

Another option is to alternate the chosen remedy with allergens (if they are known). For example, in one patient with nose and ear blockage worse in a warm room, who responded reasonably well to *Pulsatilla 30* daily, the response was better when we gave *Pulsatilla* alternating with *Mixed Pollens 12c*. After one month, the *Pulsatilla* was continued alternating with *Mixed Pollens 6c*. The lower potency is closer to the crude substance, thus it prepares the patient for exposure to the offending allergens. When using desensitising drops in this way, we potentise plants growing in the vicinity of the patient's home. This is preferable to relying on the pollen stocks from suppliers, which mostly contain European plant varieties.

[105]
Chronic Treatment:

Bacterial infection
In obstinate cases isolating a specific bacterium in potency can be effective. The most common of these is streptococcus pneumoniae, given in 10M potency twice daily for one or two weeks. Repeat in higher potencies if needed. Other bacteria to consider are: staphylococcus albus; staphylococcus aureus; streptococcus viride, streptococcus lancefield; haemophilus influenzae; klebsiella pneumoniae and neisseria catarrhalis. Also consider pseudomonas and mycoplasma.

If no swab culture has been conducted use *Sinusitis nosode, Streptococcinum and Staphylococcinum 10M* mixed.

[106]
Chronic Treatment:
Drug miasms
Penicillin and other allopathic medications can create an impediment to cure. These can be given in potency to remove the impediment. For example, Julian's proving of penicillin shows a pathogenesis of sub-febrile conditions with catarrh and right-sided sinus pain. *Penicillin 200* can be both curative, if there is a clear 'never well since' antibiotics, or it can allow the medicine of choice to act.

[107]
Summary: chronic sinusitis with *thick* yellow or green mucus
- *Kali carb 200*: Chronic sinus symptoms with asthma and allergies.
- *Tuberculinum bov 1M*: Chronic sinus symptoms where there are multiple environmental sensitivities.
- *Sanguinaria 200*: The symptom focus is the sinus headache. Chronic sinus with thick, yellow mucus with sinus headache.
- *Pyrogenium 200*: Purulent discharges. If there is a blocked ear, add *Pulsatilla 30* to the same bottle.
- *Pulsatilla 30 or 200*: Symptoms as described in the above table plus blockage of the middle ear. Mucus is either watery, watery-yellow, or yellow.
- *Mercurius sol 200*: The focus is mucous congestion and deep bone pain. Green or yellow mucus with scabs; deep pain in the facial bones; sore glands, ear ache and aggravation at night.
- *Lycopodium 30:* Blocked nose worse at night with thick elastic plugs (*Kali-b*).

[108]
Summary: chronic rhinitis with *thin* mucus
- *Kali carb 200:* Rhinitis plus asthma and allergies.
- *Tuberculinum bov 1M*: Chronic rhinitis with multiple environmental sensitivities.

- *Ammonium carb 200*: Rhinitis with sneezing, sometimes asthma, and blocked nose+++ with clear night aggravation. This is also a polyp remedy.
- *Hepar sulph 200*: Rhinitis associated with swollen lymphatic glands, sore throat and cold air sensitivity. The focus is in the throat.
- *Pulsatilla 30 or 200*: Symptoms as described in the above table plus blockage of the middle ear. Mucus is either watery, watery-yellow, or yellow.

- *Gelsemium 200:* Heavy feeling in sinuses, with sensation of dizziness, dull head and drooping eyelids.
- *Histaminum* plus allergy desensitisation: treatment option where there are only one or two allergens which produce specific symptoms, eg grass pollen in spring.
  See also the remedies in the above table for acute rhinitis and sinusitis.

Main Polychrests in Common Sinus Symptoms

Blocked nose worse at night	*Lyc, Nux, Am-c*
Post nasal discharge	*Kali-b, Nat-m, Sep, Hep-s, Nat-c, Psor, Ferr-ph*
Chronic sinusitis	*Sil, Merc, Lyc, Hydr*
Nose blockage one sided	*Nux, Sulph*

OZAENA

[109]
Clinical presentation
Ozaena is atrophic rhinitis with foul odour, anosmia, dryness and atrophy of the mucous membranes. Green crust formation, and secondary infection can occur. Dryness may be so severe that epistaxis occurs if the patient tries to remove the crust. There is often headache and nasal obstruction. Miasmatically, consider a tubercular or syphilitic remedy.

[110]
Differential diagnosis
Nasal polyps; adenoid hypertrophy; malignant ulceration; septal deviation.

Stubborn post nasal discharges may be caused by gastric reflux: there is a constant low grade irritation of the mucosa from gastric acid rising into the mouth.

[111]
Treatment
In one case, the post nasal discharge cleared up after the patient's dental amalgams were removed.

- *Aurum met 200:* Severe, deep pain in the bones of the face, with anosmia.
- *Kali bich 30 or 200:* Severe pain shooting from root of nose to external angle of eye. Use this remedy when the case relapses after having had surgical removal of polyps. (cf *Staphysagria* which has ailments following surgery).
- *Kali iod 200:* Occasional watery, acrid discharge, sometimes purulent; the nostrils may otherwise be loaded with thick, tenacious mucus (*Kali bich*). This is a syphilitic remedy: check for an actual septal perforation.
- *Nitric ac 30 or 200*: Syphilitic ulceration (particular if at muco-cutaneous junction) with bleeding.
- *Natrum mur 30***:** Consider *Natrum* whenever there is anosmia and loss of taste, or where there are obstructed lachrymal ducts resulting in ozaena with tears.
- *Syphilinum 30:* Offensive smell and red, fiery ulceration.
- *Sanguinaria 200:* Useful where frontal headache is the predominant symptom combined with yellow or green ozeana.
- In unresponsive cases, or where none of the above symptomatologies are clear, try *Pyrogenium 200* mixed with *Staphylococcus aureus 10M* and *Streptococcus pneumoniae 10M*, repeated in ascending potencies.

See Chronic Sinusitis at [102].

BRONCHITIS

[112]
Clinical presentation
Fever, chest cough: at first dry then later with purulent sputum which distresses the patient; burning chest pain < coughing; malaise. On auscultation diffuse rhonchi and moist rales can be heard. There may be wheezing after the cough.

[113]
Differential diagnosis
Adults
Asthma; pneumonia (see table at [81]). Cardiac disease (chest pain and cough). Pleurisy (chest pain without cough). Herpes zoster (surface thoracic pain without cough). Neoplasm (cough, localised absence of normal chest sounds).

Infants
Bronchiolitis.

[114]
Treatment
Adults
Where there are no clear individualising symptoms, begin with *Bryonia 30* alternating with *Kali carb 200* until there is a clear picture. These two remedies alternated are of great value in bronchitis treatment.

- *Bryonia 30 or 200:* Where there is diffuse chest pain < coughing.
- *Phosphorus 200:* Where symptoms have moved *suddenly* into the chest and the patient is rapidly weak. If this coincides with a very high fever it may be pneumonia.
- *Tuberculinum bov 1M:* Shifting symptoms, particularly if there is chest pain and pain behind the eyes. The pain moves location.
- *Kali bich 30 or 200:* If the chest pain is confined to a tiny spot. Tough, elastic phlegm.
- *Stannum met 200:* If the patient has weakness out of proportion to the illness.
- *Lycopodium 200:* Right-sided chest rhonchi with mid-afternoon aggravation.
- *Arsenicum 200:* Burning in the chest with either dyspnoea or sense of weight on the chest. Restlessness.
- *Silicea 200:* Chronic, obstinate symptoms which are unresponsive to treatment, with a marked aggravation from cold air.
- *Kali mur & Ferrum phos 3x trit:* Use in bronchitis with low fever without chest pain. Children also respond well to this remedy.
- *Causticum 200:* Sensation as though the phlegm is so deep in the chest one cannot cough deeply enough to expectorate it. Aggravation from any winds (not just cold winds).

Children
Small children are more likely to have bronchiolitis (see chart at [81]). In bronchiolitis the patient is seldom bothered by their chest cough, despite the fact that it is loud and rattling, and causes much concern to parents. NB: a very high fever with grunting on expiration suggests pneumonia, especially if there is rapid breathing or supra-sternal retraction.

- *Ipecac 30:* Works well in most cases of bronchiolitis (vomiting does not need to be a symptom).
- Alternate *Ipecac* with *Ferrum phos & Kali mur 3x trit* if there is a fever.

Summary
Adults
- *Kali carb 200 alternating with Bryonia 30:* No other remedies are clear.
- *Bryonia 30, 200:* The main remedy for diffuse chest pain < cough.
- *Phosphorus 200:* Rapid descent into the chest; aggravation from cold air.
- *Tuberculinum 1M:* Wandering symptoms with pain behind the eyes.
- *Kali bich 30/200:* Localised chest pain.
- *Stannum met 200:* Weakness out of proportion.
- *Lycopodium 200:* Right-sided rhonchi; mid afternoon aggravation.
- *Silicea 200:* Obstinate, cold cases.
- *Causticum 200:* Cannot reach the phlegm.

Children
- *Kali mur & Ferrum phos 3x trit:* Use in bronchitis with low fever without chest pain.
- *Ipecac 30:* Bronchiolitis (infants).

GLANDULAR FEVER (Infectious Mononucleosis)

[115]
Clinical presentation
Typical symptoms include painful, swollen cervical, sub-mandibular (and occasionally groin and axilla) lymph glands, pharyngitis, malaise and fever. There may be no acute episode, only unexplained malaise, which can endure for months.

Chronic glandular fever and its sequelae, are becoming more prevalent. The acute glandular pains and swellings pass, yet malaise, headache and compromised immunity result. Patients may have repeated colds, sore throats, recurring bouts of influenza, pharyngitis, laryngitis and fatigue (see [16]).

[116]
Differential diagnosis
Viral infections of the throat and glands, eg mumps (parotid glands); coxsackievirus; cytomegalovirus. Tonsillitis; pharyngitis. Chronic Fatigue Syndrome: [124] ff.

[117]
Treatment: Acute
- *Mercurius viv 200:* Where the focus of the disease is pain in the glands.
- *Belladonna 30 or 200:* If there is less glandular swelling yet nonetheless soreness, high fever, flushed appearance. This can be alternated with *Mercurius viv* if glandular pain is also prominent. At the onset of fever, before the diagnosis of glandular fever is confirmed, *Belladonna* often provides the best starting point to treatment.
- *Gelsemium 200:* If the glandular symptoms are not paramount, but malaise and headaches are prominent.
- *Ailanthus 200:* If glandular swelling persists, with low grade fever and malaise, after the acute phase should have passed, this remedy may be needed for this state of 'adynamia'.

If pharyngitis is paramount, refer to the remedies for that condition at [16]ff. Antibiotics are unnecessary and may compromise the long term recovery outcome, considering that glandular fever is a viral, not bacterial, disease.

[118]
Summary: Acute
- *Mercurius viv 200*: Swollen glands.
- *Belladonna 30, 200*: Fever.
- *Gelsemium 200*: Malaise.
- *Ailanthus 200*: 'Adynamia'.

[119]
Treatment: Chronic

Practitioners may be tempted to prescribe *Glandular Fever Nosode* but take care with this nosode, as it can aggravate. For ongoing sore throats and colds use *Coxsackievirus 30*, repeated often, which can bring about an outright cure. Where fatigue and insomnia have become established, use *Carcinosin 200*. If there is ongoing malaise and headache, *Gelsemium 200* can be repeated often until better. If there is malaise and fatigue without headache or heaviness of the head, *Kali phos 30* is preferable. For ongoing malaise and headache in children, use *Calcarea phos 200*.

[120]
Summary (chronic)
- *Coxsackievirus 30*: Colds, sore throats.
- *Carcinosin 200*: Chronic fatigue, insomnia.
- *Gelsemium 200*: Malaise, headache.
- *Kali phos 30*: Fatigue but no headache.
- *Calcarea phos 200*: Fatigue and headache in children.

CORONARY ARTERY DISEASE/ANGINA

[121]
Clinical presentation
Chest pain and breathlessness, especially when walking uphill; syncope and effort intolerance.

It is uncommon for cardiac patients to present for homeopathy. Patients who have received cardiac surgery yet still experience symptoms of pain or breathlessness are more likely to seek homeopathic support. The same medicines apply whether the patient has had cardiac surgery or not.

[122]
Differential diagnosis
Aside from other cardiac diseases: lung cancer; chronic obstructive pulmonary disease (COPD); pleurisy.

[123]
Treatment
We supplement with Vitamin E (caution for the use of vitamin E in hypertension) and Co-Enzyme Q10 for cardiovascular support. Patients should be instructed to:
o   Maintain their allopathic medication
o   Have regular blood pressure checks
o   Keep seeing their cardiologist for the stipulated check ups.

The main remedies:
- *Aconite 200*: The main remedy, which reduces chest pain and anxiety, the latter of which can compound symptoms. In some cases *Aconite* reduces a systolic hypertension.
- *Cactus 200:* Use this remedy instead of *Aconite* if the pain is constrictive.
- *Arnica 3.* In diastolic hypertension, alternate *Aconite* with *Arnica 3*.
- *Bryonia 30:* Where breathlessness is the main symptom, *Bryonia* 30 can be alternated with *Aconite 200*.

Aconite, Bryonia and Arnica can be alternated one remedy per day. One would expect to see some improvement both in pain and breathlessness within one month, even in very chronic cases. Cases which are either not operable, or have experienced no reduction in symptoms following surgery, may also benefit by referral for chelation therapy. This specialist modality is offered by some medical practitioners and has achieved some outstanding anecdotal results.

CHRONIC FATIGUE SYNDROME & FIBROMYALGIA

[124]
Clinical presentation &
Differential diagnosis
In order for a diagnosis of Chronic Fatigue Syndrome (CFS) to be made, the patient must have at least three of the following symptoms for several months:
o Extreme fatigue generally not improved by rest
o Post-exertion malaise
o Fibromyalgia
o Muscle weakness
o Impaired memory and concentration
o Insomnia
o Ongoing sore throat and tender lymph nodes
o Joint pain without inflammation
o Chronic headaches
o Dizziness.

Other symptoms associated with chronic fatigue are: Irritable Bowel Syndrome, multiple food intolerances and chemical sensitivities. A small number of patients have cold intolerance; Restless Leg Syndrome and Irritable Bladder Syndrome.
  Chronic tiredness without any other of the above symptoms should not be diagnosed as CFS. There are other causes of tiredness which should be investigated. Some red flag symptoms may suggest a more sinister diagnosis. These are: weight loss; fever; persistent malaise; night pain; focal pain and neurological signs. The following are *not* CFS:
o *Anaemia:* Check colour of eyelids and nails or refer for iron and haemoglobin studies. Check vitamin B12 deficiency, especially in vegetarians.
o *Hepatic disease:* Sluggish bile flow can cause fatigue, while in advanced liver disease, eg fatty liver or cirrhosis, other signs will appear, such as intolerance to fatty food, thirst, etc. Refer for liver function test.
o *Diabetes:* Symptoms alone can be strongly suggestive even without medical tests. Check for weight loss, nocturia, dry mouth, excessive thirst, appetite changes, visual disturbance, susceptibility to infection and history of boils. Examine the urine and refer for a glucose tolerance test.
o *Hypoglycaemia:* Dizziness, headache or vagueness between meals, unusual sweating, palpitations (can be confused with anxiety), tremor, irritability, excessive hunger and tachycardia (cf cardiac disease). Refer for glucose tolerance test. These symptoms can be confused with GIT candida. See [46].
o *Kidney disease:* Refer for urea and creatinine tests and urine culture for urinary tract infection (UTI). Check blood pressure.
o *Malnutrition:* Despite a Western diet, malnutrition still poses a problem. Check vitamin B12 status in vegetarians plus iron and haemaglobin, especially in menstruating women.
o *Infection:* Chronic low grade infection such as urinary tract infection (UTI); slow tooth abcess; tonsillitis; Pelvic Inflammatory Disease.

o *Intestinal parasites:* A child who has symptoms of intermittent abdominal pain around the umbilicus, itchy rectum or nose, nocturnal teeth grinding, variable appetite, failure to thrive or unexplained headaches, should be referred for stool analysis.
o *Cancer:* Fatigue plus unexplained weight loss could suggest malignancy. Referral is needed if the patient is unresponsive to homeopathic treatment.
o *Lifestyle:* Stress, lack of sleep and exercise and poor diet are common causes of chronic tiredness.
o *Mental illness:* Check for signs of depression, agoraphobia or anxiety and make the appropriate referrals.
o *Insomnia or sleep apnoea:* A chronic snorer (child or adult) may have sleep apnoea. Apnoea may be caused by adenoid hypertrophy, nasal polyps or ozeana, obesity or cardiac disease.
o *Hypothyroidism:* Weight gain, loss of hair, brittle nails, palpitations.

Fibromyalgia
CFS patients frequently have fibromyalgia. Symptoms include:
o Generalised muscle pain with tender points
o Paresthesia
o Skin sensitivity
o Temporo-mandibular joint dysfunction.
Although fibromyalgia is a separate syndrome from CFS, it is included here because it is commonly associated with CFS.

[125]
Aetiology
The aetiology in CFS is often a challenge to orthodox medicine. Possibilities are viral, psychological, genetic predisposition, allergic and history of exposure to chemical toxins. Although viral causes are postulated, there is no evidence that CFS is contagious. In recent years there has been discussion of 'stealth viruses' where no specific viral pathogen is found at all, yet viral indicators appear in pathology tests.

'Classical' CFS commonly begins with a viral episode like influenza or glandular fever, with symptoms of sore throat, fever, muscle pain and weakness.

With so many disparate presenting symptoms, CFS and fibromyalgia present a management challenge for any health professional.

Because of this complexity, range and individuality of symptoms, homeopathy is well placed to provide effective treatment.

The following categories are not mutually exclusive. An emotional aetiology can be the fuel for an allergic diathesis or a post-viral syndrome. Careful case-taking and diagnostic tests (eg heavy metal toxicity) are essential to find the aetiology in this syndrome. *The most important question to ask is 'When did it start?'* This is the best guide to the aetiology.

Treatment

This treatment section is divided into the following categories according to causation:

o *[126] Post viral*
o *[127] Allergy or sensitivity*
o *[128] Emotional*
o *[129] Chemical & heavy metal toxicity*
o *[130] Unknown aetiology*
o *[131] Candidiasis*
o *[132] Children*
o *[133] Hormonal*

[126]
Post viral
When a CFS patient is 'never well since' a particular virus, that virus can be given in potency with caution: it can cause aggravation. The most common of these is the Epstein Barr virus, the pathogen which is implicated in glandular fever.
* *Carcinosin 30 or 200:* Take one dose every second day if no other medicine is indicated. Fastidiousness and insomnia are keynotes. There is a family history of cancer or diabetes. The patient may have contracted a childhood disease (eg whooping cough) as an adult.
* *Gelsemium 200:* Stupor, heaviness, dullness, dizziness, trembling, weakness, muscle ache.
* Where the patient experiences continued laryngitis or pharyngitis *Coxsackievirus 30* is often beneficial: even if the symptoms date from having had glandular fever.
* In other cases, a similar virus (not the same virus) can be given in potency, since *similia* is less likely to aggravate than isopathy (see discussion below).
* *Sarcolactic Acid 200c*: extreme prostration.

Many persons with glandular fever-type symptoms, may test positive to past exposure to glandular fever without knowing they ever had the disease.
  It is possible that there is a viral causation of other symptoms associated with CFS. For example, a viral infection may precede the onset of multiple allergies or chemical sensitivity. It is important to choose a remedy based on the symptom picture, as well as a remedy based on causation. For example, a patient who has never been well since glandular fever may respond well to the *Glandular Fever Nosode,* yet their symptoms may only be partially addressed by that remedy. It is safer to give a traditional remedy based on the symptom picture first, such as *Gelsemium* (described below) to initiate improvement before giving the patient the same (as opposed to similar) pathogen. In our example of glandular fever, if one chooses a **similar** pathogen, such as *Coxsackievirus*, rather than Glandular fever nosode, there may be a better patient response with less likelihood of aggravation.

[127]
Allergy or sensitivity

An identifiable allergy must be isolated and the offending substance removed from the patient's environment (whether internal or external) if possible. This may include food, pollens and household or industrial chemicals. The difference between allergies and sensitivities and the methods for testing allergy and sensitivity are discussed at [89] ff. Failure to isolate and remove an allergen from the patient's environment creates an *obstacle to cure*.

Common food allergens are: dairy, yeast, wheat, crustaceans, salicylates, and sometimes amines. A patient with no previous history of allergy can develop allergic reactions in his/her state of illness. The offending allergens are still best removed during treatment. When the patient is well a challenge test can then be given and the substance permitted provided there is no reaction.

Food sensitivities (as opposed to allergies) are in the same category and must be eliminated from the diet until the patient has improved. In this age, everyone has ingested antibiotics. It is well known that antibiotics cause altered bowel flora which can lead to gut dysbiosis. In a case of multiple food sensitivities associated with CFS or other systemic symptoms such as weakness, multiple histamine responses (itch; urticaria; sneezing; coryza etc) together with functional disturbances such as unexplained insomnia, headaches etc, it is very difficult to find a causation, let alone an accurate diagnosis. It is wise in these cases to commence treatment with a bowel nosode. The genius of bowel nosodes is that chronic cases can respond quickly: sometimes after only one dose. We repeat the bowel nosode in the 30th potency daily until there is a favourable reaction (or aggravation). If a favourable reaction occurs, then reduce the nosode to every second day. Stop the remedy on aggravation, then re-assess the case, taking careful note of any new symptoms.

In every case, one must be able to discern an improvement (even if small) on a general level, *even though the particular symptoms may change*. For example, a slight reduction in headaches or insomnia is a positive sign, even if a new *particular* symptom arises. This is in keeping with Hering's Law. If the new symptom is strong enough to cause discomfort, suspend chronic treatment and use an acute remedy as needed, then return to the chronic treatment. However, it is best not to interrupt the treatment in this way unless it is absolutely essential. The ground you have gained in vitality of the patient will often remain slippery.

Paterson's treatise on bowel nosodes (see Bibliography) is the most user-friendly, since it gives a table of comparative materia medica. There are often useful keynotes to aid in their selection. For example:

- *Morgan Gaertner 30:* If the patient has a history of gallbladder disease, OR their stool colour is pale OR s/he experiences nausea after fat or rich food (suggesting poor bile flow).
- *Morgan (Bach) 30:* Where there is eczema or asthma as part of the symptomatology.

The relationship between the bowel and immune function has been discussed briefly at [38] ff. This relationship cannot be overestimated in the treatment of chronic disease in adults. Similarly, general disturbances, such as anxiety, irritability, insomnia, may all be improved by bowel nosodes.

Below are some of the key words we use to aid choosing a bowel nosode:

Bowel Nosodes: Key words

Alternation of symptoms	Mutabile
Anticipatory anxiety	Dysentery Co
Asthma alternates with eczema	Mutabile
Avoids company	Morgan (Bach); Morgan Pure
Congestion & sluggishness	Morgan (Bach)
Criticism, highly sensitive to	Dysentery Co
Depressive	Morgan (Bach)
Eczema in children	Morgan (Bach)
Emaciation & malnutrition	Gaertner (Bach)
Fatigue – feels unfit for the task	Bacillus #7
Fidgety, shy	Dysentery Co
Hypersensitive – brain overactive	Gaertner (Bach)
Hysteria	Proteus (Bach)
Introspection	Morg (Bach)
Irritability	Sycotic Co
Nerve strain – brain storm	Proteus (Bach)
Spasm – neurological	Proteus (Bach)
Sudden onset	Proteus (Bach)
Violent outburst with kicking & screaming	Proteus (Bach)

©Jon Gamble 2004

[128]
Emotional

Stress or emotional issues may be a part of the CFS spectrum. In one case a young man with multiple food sensitivities and exhaustion, was certain that his disease began after the death of his mother. He blamed his father's mistreatment of his mother for her death Because of this he hated his father. A single dose of *Natrum carb 200* completely cured the case because the causation was clearly identifiable (ie grief as causation with hatred of one particular family member). In many cases one can discern an underlying and pre-existing anxiety, and there may be issues within the family which need resolution. Referral for counselling is recommended in these cases. An underlying chronic anxiety may precede the onset of CFS.

Remedy possibilities are endless when there is an emotional causation of CFS. Some of these are:
• *Ignatia 200*: Symptoms do not add up; for example she only gets the pain when she walks in a certain street. The patient is emotionally on the edge with easy tears and frequent sighing. Symptoms always come when she is

stressed. No emotional equilibrium. The patient may be unable to point to the precise symptoms.

- *Natrum mur 200:* The symptoms began with a sudden loss or grief. Or the patient can never forgive what has happened. Emotional pain is nonetheless concealed. S/he feels separate from the world, yet may be quietly superior.
- *Natrum carb 200*: As for *Natrum mur* but s/he has a particular dislike of one person, usually a family member, whom s/he cannot forgive: s/he regards them as being responsible for the grief. (See the case described in the above paragraph.)
- *Carcinosin 30 or 200*: The patient was overly responsible as a child, became a vicarious parent by assuming responsibility for the family's wellbeing. May have Obsessive-Compulsive Disorder, a history of insomnia or a family history of cancer or diabetes. *Carcinosin* has a wide field in the treatment of CFS even in the absence of the traditional mentals of *Carcinosin*. Foubister gives a well-rounded description of *Carcinosin*. See the Bibliography.
- *Thuja 200*: There is deep shame, which may surround an event such as rape or long term emotional abuse, where the victim feels they were partly responsible for the incident.

Patients in this category will benefit from counselling concurrently with homeopathic treatment.

[129]
Chemical & heavy metal toxicity

Chemical toxicity can be determined by a variety of tests. Simple urine tests can determine the presence of heavy metals. Acu-dermal testing and applied kinesiology can also assess chemical toxicity. However, hair mineral analysis probably gives us the most accurate assessment. One pointer to the possibility of chemical toxicity, is the presence of a physical pathology with the CFS. (CFS is usually a purely functional disease.) For example, in a CFS case of alopecia and crumbling fingernails the patient's hair analysis showed lead toxicity. A patient suffering from dermatitis which was unresponsive to the usual treatments returned a hair analysis for mercury toxicity.

To enhance elimination of heavy metals, the product homeopathic complex 'CH-77' is a useful starting point. This is an aklalising complex which facilitates chelation of heavy metals. It contains alkalizing minerals in low potency:

- *Potassium chloride 5x*
- *Sodium bicarbonate 5x*
- *Magnesium sulphate 5x*
- *Citric acid 5x.*

However when a specific metal is isolated, that metal can be given in high potency. This should be supported with liver drainage, or kidney drainage in some cases. Use herbal tinctures such as *Chelidonium, Berberis and Dandelion* in mother tincture or 1x. Where one particular heavy metal is identified, that heavy metal can be given in the 200th potency if symptoms agree. This can be given weekly for many weeks.

Any toxic mineral can result in chronic fatigue. Here are common symptoms of crude poisoning:

Toxic Minerals	Symptoms
Arsenic.	GIT: burning, diarrhoea; dyspnoea; anxiety
Cadmium.	Headache; dyspnoea; diarrhoea; GIT cramps
Aluminium.	Constipation, nausea, appetite loss; twitching limbs; fatigue; difficulty in concentration
Lead.	Encephalopathy; anaemia; colic; hyperactivity, learning disorders in children
Mercury.	GIT burning; skin irritations; diseases characterized by ulceration.*

*In my opinion mercury toxicity predisposes to melanoma in susceptible patients.

In addition to specific heavy metals, the residual pesticides of *DDT, dieldrin* and *heptachlor* were only banned in Australia some 20 years ago. These chemicals travel the world in water vapour and are dumped whenever it rains. Other sources are found in food, eg mercury in offshore fish. *Constitutionally susceptible patients absorb and retain traces of these chemicals, no matter where they live or what they eat.* Patients who are not constitutionally susceptible are still at risk if they were exposed to large enough doses of these chemicals.

[130]
Unknown aetiology
Different aetiologies may combine to produce CFS. *In some cases no amount of investigation can determine any aetiology whatsoever.* Constitutional prescribing is essential in these cases, which may include the 'emotional' medicines listed above.

A viral pathogen in potency can be alternated with a traditional homeopathic medicine, can give better initial results, as mentioned above.

- *Toxoplasmosis 30 or 200:* When fibromyalgia is a pronounced symptom, use *Toxoplasmosis 30 or 200*. Toxoplasmosis is usually contracted from eating meat which is not properly cooked. In chronic cases of toxoplasmosis infection the pathogen causes abnormal muscle fatigue, bowel disturbance – usually diarrhoea, painful flatulence, and major food sensitivities. Its pathogenesis therefore has a clear application for these types of chronic fatigue syndrome with fibromyalgia. *Toxoplasmosis* can be alternated with a constitutional medicine.

- *Gelsemium 200 and Toxoplasmosis 200*: Prescribe on alternate days for steady results.
- *Carcinosin:* As described at [128].
- *Scutellaria 200*: Weakness plus anxiety and dullness.
- *Helleborus 200*: Stupefaction: where the senses are functioning but the brain processes nothing: eg one hears the words but has difficulty understanding them.
- *Baptisia 200*: Severe muscle pain and stupor.

[131]
Candidiasis
Ingestion of too many sugars and carbohydrates combined with overuse of antibiotics and stress can result in GIT candida. In some patients, use of the oral contraceptive pill predisposes to candida. See the section on Candida at [46] ff.

[132]
Children
CFS in children is becoming more prevalent. Aetiologies in these children are largely unknown. Glandular fever is relatively common in teenagers. See [126].

One of the most common presenting symptoms in children with CFS is severe ongoing headache, coupled with fibromyalgia and poor sleep patterns. These children respond well to *Calcarea phos 200* every second day. Supplementation with mineral doses of calcium and magnesium phosphate assists sleep and reduces fibromyalgia. All the 'adult' remedies can also be used in children.

[133]
Treatment:
Hormonal
Ongoing fatigue, dizziness, foggy head, anxiety, fibromyalgia, may also be caused by taking synthetic oestrogen as in the oral contraceptive pill (or HRT). Ask female patients if the symptom onset coincided with starting, or changing, the contraceptive pill. If so, the pill should be withdrawn and the patient prescribed *Folliculinum 30* for weeks to months. See also Oestrogen Dominance at [56].

[134]
Summary
Most frequently used medicines in CFS of unknown or post viral aetiology:
- *Carcinosin 30, 200*: for CFS patients with the typical *Carcinosin* history or family history (see Foubister in the Bibliography); or when no other remedy is indicated. Keynotes are insomnia and fastidiousness.
- *Gelsemium 200:* stupor, heaviness, dullness, dizziness, trembling, weakness, muscle ache and headache.

These medicines can be alternated with one of the following pathogenetic medicines:

- *Toxoplasmosis 30 or 200:* Fibromyalgia.
- *Coxsackievirus 30:* Recurring pharyngitis.
- *Glandular fever 30:* (With caution) where never well since glandular fever.

These remedies may either cure or improve symptoms, giving us time to work out the patient's constitutional medicine.

- *Bowel nosodes:* For multiple food sensitivities and Irritable Bowel Syndrome.

Other medicines which have been found effective in CFS:

- *Calcarea phos 200*: In children with debilitating headache, sometimes nausea, as primary symptom.
- *Folliculinum 30*: Side effects from synthetic oestrogen (ie iatrogenic cause).

GASTRITIS, PEPTIC ULCER & INDIGESTION

[135]
Clinical presentation
Epigastric pain, heartburn, eructations with or without burning, hoarse voice, laryngeal irritation, cough or mucus, regurgitation or sensation of a lump in the throat unexplained by other causes.

[136]
Differential diagnosis
Gastric neoplasm; oesophagitis; Barrett's oesophagus; pyloric stenosis; disease of the gallbladder (including stasis); scleroderma of the oesophagus; polyps of the vocal chords; post-nasal drip; hyperchlorhydria.

[137]
Treatment
There are different presentations of gastritis and indigestion as described below.

[138]
Treatment:
With reflux
- *Robinia 3:* In heartburn and reflux, where the burning sensation extends from the stomach up into the oesophagus. Sour burping. The pain occurs some time after eating. Mix with *Natrum phos 3x trit* for good results. In chronic cases, this can be repeated for months.
- *Abies nig 6:* A sensation of a lump in the *top* of the stomach (ie, cardiac orifice) 'as if he had swallowed an egg'.
- *Arsenicum 3:* Severe epigastric pain immediately after eating, with vomiting which then relieves the pain. Do not use *Arsenicum* if there is haematemesis.
- *Lycopodium 30 or 200:* Abundant flatulence. The flatus itself may cause reflux because of the pressure it places on the stomach and pylorus.
- *Ignatia 200*: Reflux with minimal or no pain: merely a sensation of lump in the throat, or sometimes a scratchy larynx.
- *Nux vom 30*: This remedy is specific for retro-sternal pain with reflux, of the type commonly found in hiatus hernia.
- *Asafoetida 6*: Hysteric belching with heartburn < thinking about it.

[139]
Treatment:
Without reflux
Where there is no reflux, and pain is confined to the epigastric region:
- *Chelidonium 30*: Poor appetite and pain, yet the pain is improved by eating.
- *Anacardium 200*: Where there is good appetite, and the pain is also improved by eating.
- *Arsenicum 3* can also be used for epigastric pain, where there is no reflux. Aggravation occurs immediately after food, which is relieved by vomiting.

[140]
Treatment:
Peptic ulcers
Ulceration can be treated with any of the above remedies, depending on the presenting symptoms. The most common prescription is:
- *Arsenicum 3* alternated with *Anacardium 200* on alternate days. This yields excellent results. Patients report great improvement after two weeks.

The current trend of using antibiotic therapy to kill *helicobacter pylori* is unnecessary if the correct homeopathic remedy is chosen, together with appropriate dietary considerations.

In chronic gastritis, a bland diet is not advised, since stomach enzymes and hydrochloric acid in *most* cases need to be **stimulated**, not suppressed. Allopathic reasoning, unfortunately, is that stomach juices need to be alkalised. This is the opposite of what is needed for most patients who are no better after many years on antacid medication if they stop the medicine. **Many cases of gastritis and reflux respond well to the protocols for treating hypochlorhydria**. For a full discussion see Hypochlorhydria at [142].

When patients stop their antacid medication, rebound symptoms can occur. These are well managed with half teaspoon of bicarb soda in a little water, which quickly relieves heartburn.

Another factor in some patients is poor intestinal peristalsis. Although a patient may have regular bowel movements, there may be incomplete emptying. In other words, there is a stasis of the intestinal system, which is a contributing factor in reflux by exerting pressure upwards onto the cardiac sphincter. These patients often respond well to:
- *Nux vom 30*, repeated every second day. *Nux* will improve both the gastritis and the poor bowel function. The usual modalities and mental characteristics do not need to be present for *Nux* to be effective. The pain in *Nux* is generally felt in the oesophagus.

Please note that while most patients with gastritis and indigestion need stomach acid stimulation, a small number do not. Read the section on Hypochlorhydria at [142] before proceeding.

Summary
Main treatment for peptic ulcer:
- *Arsenicum 3:* two doses on one day, alternating with *Anacardium 200* on the alternate day, continued for many weeks to months in chronic cases.

[141]
Treatment options for gastritis of more obscure causes
(a) Scleroderma
In scleroderma the oesophagus and pyloric sphincter develop a stricture or the classic 'hidebound' pathology described for scleroderma, in which case *Hepar sulph 6* is more effective than the above remedies.

(b) Biliary calculi
Biliary calculi or simple gall sludge can cause reflux and heartburn, as well as acute colic in cholecystitis. See that section for treatments at [144].

(c) Globus hystericus
This is somaticised anxiety: the patient experiences a lump in the throat with a feeling of suffocation or breathlessness. Whenever a patient complains of a sensation of a lump in the throat, make sure it is only a sensation. Inspect for glandular swellings, including enlarged thyroid.
- *Ignatia 200*: The main remedy for *globus hystericus.*
- *Argentum nit 200:* For *globus* plus clear claustrophobia (cannot go into a tunnel).
- *Asafoetida 6:* tension, anxiety in stomach with forcible belching < thinking about it.

(d) Heavy metal or mineral toxicity
Arsenic toxicity in particular will cause gastritis. See the discussion of heavy metals in CFS at [129].

(e) Coeliac disease
Persistent indigestion and heartburn may be caused by undiagnosed coeliac disease, particularly if there is diarrhoea as well. Removal of gluten from the diet is essential once diagnosis has been confirmed by pathology.

HYPOCHLORHYDRIA

[142]
Clinical presentation &
Overview
See the symptoms and differential diagnoses described for Gastritis, Peptic ulcer & Indigestion at [135] ff.

Acidity, heartburn, bloating and reflux are common symptoms in hypochlorhydria.

It is important to determine the presence or not of hypochlorhydria (insufficient hydrochloric acid of the stomach) in gastritis, indigestion, reflux, colic, etc, since this will influence the prescription and dietary advice. *Hypochlorhydria is far more common than hyperchlorhydria,* yet it is unacknowledged in conventional medicine. The reasons why hypochlorhydria causes gastritis and heartburn are unclear.

To determine the presence or not of hypochlorhydria, there are some reliable signs:
- Patient describes a sense of heaviness, fullness or coldness immediately having eaten. The food sits heavily and there is burping soon afterwards.
- *The tongue:* A white or grey tongue will suggest insufficient acid, while a thick creamy yellow tongue suggests over-acidity.

[143]
Treatment
Treatment of hypochlorhydria necessitates a diet which will stimulate HCl, even where there is gastritis or dyspepsia. Patients may think that stimulation of their stomach acid is the wrong approach, since they have been told for years that they have too much acid. Unfortunately, their treatment may have managed, but has not improved, the condition.

Over-indulgence in refined carbohydrates, stress, greasy take-away foods and pre-packaged convenience food are all factors which contribute to disturbance in HCl. These foods, especially refined carbohydrates, should be discouraged. Many patients with hypochlorhydria cannot tolerate tomato-based products.

Treatment for stomach acid imbalance is very important as it affects the whole gastrointestinal system, and has rebound effects on other body systems.

Avoid bland diets. Any of the aromatic culinary herbs, ie curries with turmeric, cardamom, cumin etc, will stimulate HCl. A small amount of hot chilli can be homeopathic, but be careful, especially in the case of gastric ulcer, as it may aggravate. If a small amount can be tolerated, it should be encouraged. The patient should not consume liquid before meals, as this further dilutes the HCl. The patient should drink only when thirsty, and not conform to what is considered 'the right amount' to drink. It is better to drink between meals.

Lemon juice and apple cider vinegar both stimulate stomach acid, and can be taken before and/or after meals in a little water. Patients with severe reflux may not tolerate apple cider vinegar, so this should be used with caution.

See treatment options in Gastritis, Peptic ulcer & Indigestion at [135]. The following two remedies are reliable in commencing treatment.

Hypochlorhydria:
- *Gentian MT:* For hypochlorhydria, give gentian mother tincture, 15 drops in a little water 20 minutes before food, to stimulate HCl. If this causes heartburn, take it immediately before meals, until it no longer causes heartburn; then return to the 20 minute gap before meals.
- *Chelidonium MT:* In many cases of stomach acid disturbance, especially where diet has been particularly poor as described above, the bile flow is poor. The patient has pale stools, nausea, afternoon headaches and intolerance to fat or greasy food. *Chelidonium* mother tincture: 15-20 drops in water 20 minutes before meals. *Chelidonium* can be mixed with *Gentian* if both remedies are indicated. The dose in this case is 20-25 drops per dose.
- If the patient experiences gastritis, reflux or indigestion, see the remedies recommended at [137].

For hyperacidity with stomach pain or oesophageal reflux, see Gastritis, Peptic ulcer & Indigestion at [135] ff.

Hyperchlorhydria:
- *Natrum phos 3x trit:* For **hyperchlorhydria** (excess stomach acid.) Combine with *Kali mur 3x* where the tongue is especially coated with grey or white. This can be given three times daily.

GALLBLADDER STASIS

[144]
Clinical presentation
Nausea alone or nausea with indigestion and possibly afternoon headache. In gallbladder calculi, there may be dull or acute pain in the epigastrium or right hypochondria, which may radiate to the right scapula.

[145]
Differential diagnosis
Gallstones can cause acute colic (cholecystitis) as well as gastric reflux, heartburn and flatulence. Indigestion, gastritis or oesophagitis. If nausea is the only symptom: check for pregnancy.

Treatment
[146]
Gallstones
To remove gallbladder stones, we use this protocol:
- *Cholesterinum 1M*: Take twice daily for three to four weeks to 'soften' the stones. Next, the patient can do a traditional lemon/olive oil cleanse. One to one and a half litres of equal parts of olive oil and lemon juice are swallowed over a four hour period, whilst fasting from solid food.

This procedure flushes many stones, including large ones. There is a concern that stones may lodge in the bile duct during this cleanse. Whilst this concern is legitimate, it has never happened in our experience, as we have witnessed very large (over 1cm) stones being easily passed with this method.

Persistent gall pain can be treated with the following remedies repeated regularly for at least 12 months and may also result in stones passing. A low-fat diet with exclusion of eggs is necessary, and daily vigorous walking encouraged.
- *China 6*: Constant pain in the right hypochondria with intermittent acute colic. For women with a recent history of childbirth, especially if still lactating.
- *Lycopodium 200*: Gallstones with constipation. Also use in asymptomatic gallstones.
- *Carduus mar 30*: Acute epigastric pain unrelated to eating. Gallbladder colic may occur every few months from gall stones.
- *Chelidonium 30:* Epigastric pain worse empty stomach. There is poor appetite. The pain may radiate to the right scapula.

[147]
Gall sludge
Sludge of the biliary duct is very common. Patients will have had ultrasounds which show no gallstones, yet they remain sensitive to greasy or fatty food with nausea and fatigue. Gallsludge is removed by giving mother tincture of *Chelidonium*, 15-20 drops in water 20 minutes three times daily before each meal, for four to eight weeks.

IRRITABLE BOWEL SYNDROME (IBS)

[148]
Clinical presentation &
Overview
Shifting abdominal pain with alternating constipation and diarrhoea, often with incomplete feeling after evacuation. The cause of IBS is unknown.

Once more serious pathologies have been ruled out, IBS remains at the bottom of the diagnostic barrel. While the patient is relieved to hear there is nothing sinister detected, allopathic treatment options offer them little more than daily use of psyllium husks or other dietary fibre.

IBS can also be a stress-related functional disturbance, eg, the bowels are fine on the weekend, but disturbed during the working week. Thus mental and emotional factors need to be considered.

Normal food sensitivity tests may fail to locate food intolerances. See the range of tests described at [89].

The most common food sensitivities are wheat, yeast, dairy and salicylates.

Excluding food sensitivities is a popular but only partial solution. Patient compliance varies. Without correct treatment, the list of sensitivities can just increase over time.

Coeliac Disease
Coeliac disease often presents with symptoms like IBS and can go undiagnosed for many years, during which an array of ineffective treatments is given. Coeliac disease can now be accurately diagnosed with appropriate pathology tests. By the time the patient reaches the homeopath, coeliac disease may already have been excluded by pathology tests. If not, referral for a test is recommended. If the patient has coeliac disease, all grains containing gluten must be excluded.

[149]
Differential diagnosis
Crohn's Disease; Ulcerative Colitis; Coeliac Disease. Presence of blood in faeces must always be investigated. Bright blood indicates rectal bleeding and is most often caused by haemorrhoids. If malignancy is suspected refer the patient for faecal occult blood test. One should also suspect a more sinister pathology in the presence of anaemia, weight loss and fevers. See Gallbladder stasis [144]; Gastritis, Peptic ulcer & Indigestion [135]; and the discussion on food sensitivities [103].

Treatment
Many patients with IBS improve with dietary changes, especially if wheat is excluded. Wheat and sugar saturate the modern western diet. Spelt, kamut or other non-wheat flours can be used in place of wheat flour.

[150]
Treatment:
Inadequate peristaltic action
* *Nux vom 30:* Where peristaltic action is inadequate, and a full evacuation is seldom achieved, even though the bowels move each day Patients may report that although they pass some stool at least once per day, they never feel as though the evacuation is complete. 'Unsatisfactory stool' is often diagnosed as IBS. Repeat *Nux* every second day.

[151]
Treatment:
Constipation
* *Bryonia 200:* The most common remedy in constipation, especially if the stool is large and dry. There may be pain at the right hypochondria. Repeated every second day, *Bryonia* cures many obstinate cases.
* *Plumbum 200:* Can be alternated with *Bryonia* on alternate days if there is no response with *Bryonia* alone.
* *Alumina 200:* The preferred remedy in extremes of age where the stool is soft.
* *Nux vom 30:* 'Never completely done' feeling, even with daily bowel movements.
* *Morgan (Bach) 200:* in chronic cases, intercurrent doses of this nosode are useful.

[152]
Treatment:
Diarrhoea
A high fibre diet in the wrong constitution, a change of diet or too much fruit, will all produce diarrhoea.
* *Podophyllum 200:* The main remedy. Loose watery stools with rumbling abdomen and slight pain.
* *Aloes 200:* Minimal pain but the patient is unsure if s/he is passing only flatus or stool, and can thus end up inadvertently soiling themselves.
* *Mercurius cor 30:* Diarrhoea associated with abdominal cramps.

Other possibilities in diarrhoea: intestinal parasites including Giardia; coeliac disease; ulcerative colitis; Crohn's disease, rotavirus in children.

[153]
Treatment:
Flatulence
Flatulence can cause pain in IBS, since it stretches the bowel wall. Having excluded possible food sensitivities, *Lycopodium 30 or 200* is the most often prescribed medicine. If the patient has a history of thrush, then the flatulence may be a symptom of GIT candidiasis: see [46] ff.

Check for sluggish liver function (eg pale stool and poor absorption of fats) or biliary stasis – see [144]; Hypochlorhydria [142]. Also check for ulcerative colitis, Crohn's disease, and coeliac disease: some of these cases still slip through the allopathic diagnostic net. Flatulence, thrush and sugar sensitivity imply GIT candida [46] ff.

[154]
Treatment:
Emotional
An emotional aetiology may be an important factor in IBS but may not be the only one. Any functional disturbance is aggravated during times of stress.
- *Ignatia 200:* The main remedy: the patient's symptoms do not quite add up. For example, as part of the IBS they experience cramping of the feet, for which there is no anatomical or physiological rationale.
- *Lycopodium 200:* The other remedy to consider is *Lycopodium*, where there is lack of self confidence hidden under a veneer of perfectionism, irritability or 'keeping up appearances'.

[155]
Treatment:
Parasitic
Giardia, cryptosporidium, clostridium difficile and entamoeba hystolytica can cause ongoing symptoms of IBS in susceptible children and adults. These pathogens can be a major cause of IBS, since they can trigger all the above categories of IBS symptoms, including emotional disturbance.
IBS caused by intestinal parasites, may have one or more of these symptoms:
- Disturbed sleep (for no apparent reason)
- Nocturnal fevers
- Restless leg syndrome
- Ongoing unexplained diarrhoea
- Recurring colds or flues (which they describe as 'allergies')
- Unexplained weakness or fatigue
- Offensive flatulence
- Abdominal pain.

Having had a stool analysis one can prescribe the intestinal pathogen in high potency (at least 20M) intercurrently with the medicine of choice. This reduces susceptibility to the organism. However, the following remedies are more effective than isopathic prescriptions:
- *Cina 200*: Where there is rectal itch, teeth grinding, nose itch, excessive irritability. Repeat two or three times weekly for at least one month.
- *Stannum 200 alternating with Nux vom 30:* Where there is persistent pain around the umbilicus, prescribe one dose on a daily basis alternating (ie approximately three doses of each per week) for one to two months. This will also improve irregularity of the bowel motions or a 'not quite done' feeling after evacuation.

For discussion of IBS in children see Abdominal Pain in Children at [24]. See *Mastering Homeopathy 2: The Treatment of Irritable Bowel Syndrome* (2006).

DISEASES OF THE SKIN

HERPES

[156]
Clinical presentation
In simplex (HSV-1 or HSV-2): small, painful vesicles which contain serous fluid appear. After a few days the vesicles form crusts. Simplex 1 often appears on or around the lips. Simplex 2 appears on, in or around the genitals or rectum. In zoster, severe pain precedes, or replaces, the eruptions. In zoster, a common (but not exclusive) site is the thoracic area, as eruptions follow a main nerve path.
  In both simplex and zoster, fever and malaise may occur.

Treatment

[157]
Shingles (herpes zoster)
If there is typical shingles-type pain but there have not been any cutaneous eruptions, the diagnosis may need revision. It may be a case of impingement of thoracic spinal nerves in which case referral for chiropractic or osteopathic manipulation is necessary. Also consider cardiac pain.
* *Arsenicum 200 alternating with Hypericum 200:* For shingles of the intercostal area. In chronic cases, continue on alternate days for some months.
* *Prunus spinosa 200:* This is specific for zoster of the intraocular nerve (where severe pain is felt in the eye).
* For zoster of the trigeminal nerve give either *Hypericum 200* (shooting pain) or *Spigelia 200* (left sided pain).
* *Cadmium sulph 30*: For zoster with distortion of mouth or inability to close the eye.
* *Zincum met 30*: Post-zoster twitching.

[158]
Simplex (HSV-1 & -2)
Check the patient's nutritional status, especially their zinc, since herpes is generally an opportunistic infection, often emerging when the patient is under stress and their immunity is compromised.
* *Nitric ac 200:* Any lesions occurring at a muco-dermal junction.
* *Arsenicum 200 alternating with Antimony crud 6:* For cold sores at the lips.
* *Arsenicum 200 alternating with Mercurius sol 200: Mercurius* has specificity for the genitalia.
* *Rhus tox 30:* Small, clear vesicles which are very itchy.
* *Natrum mur 30:* We have experienced mixed results using *Natrum mur* in acute stages and found the above remedies better.

ACNE

[159]
Clinical presentation
Blackheads; follicular pustules; deep nodules and cysts which fail to discharge the purulent matter. Deep pustules may cause scarring. Most common in puberty, it occurs on the face, shoulders, neck and back.

[160]
Treatment
The use of long term antibiotics for acne treatment disturbs gut function. Candida overgrowth of the gut, for example, may actually make acne worse. Low zinc status may predispose to acne, since low levels result in an increase in the conversion of testosterone to dihydrotestosterone. Zinc supplementation is therefore recommended.

Hormonal
Acne related to the menstrual cycle:
- *Folliculinum 30*: Women who are or have been using the oral contraceptive pill should use an alternative method of contraception, and be given *Folliculinum 30* for several weeks. This removes the synthetic oestrogens and improves the acne.
- *Sepia 200*: When acne is aggravated premenstrually and improves after the menses. Particularly indicated if there is dysmenorrhoea or menorrhagia.

Teenage
- *Kali brom 30*: Useful for teenagers who are stressed by over-studying, drink too much coke, and do not sleep well. The acne is usually found on the face and shoulders. Restricting soft drinks and other refined sugars will improve treatment results.
- *Aurum 200*: For acne of either sex confined to the face or shoulders. Also well indicated for teenagers.
- *Hepar sulph 200*: Painful, pustular acne.
- *Antimony crud 200*: Small pointed lesions.
- *Bowel nosodes*: If there is gut disturbance, especially after antibiotic use, consider one of the bowel nosodes, such as *Morgan (Bach)*.

Acne Rosacea
- *Folliculinum 30*: As mentioned above, if there has been use of the contraceptive pill, start with *Folliculinum 30*, which can later be increased to 200. An alternative method of contraception should be used. The use of synthetic oestrogens can promote acne rosacea in susceptible patients. In many cases, this will improve, and occasionally cure, rosacea.

- *Causticum 200 alternating with Antimony crud 6*: We have seen reasonable results with these remedies, bearing in mind that Rosacea is a stubborn disease.

[161]
Summary
- *Folliculinum 30:* Use of the Pill (OCD). Acne is worse at menses.
- *Sepia 200:* Acne is worse at menses plus dysmenorrhoea or menorrhagia.
- *Aurum 200*: The main remedy: a good place to start for facial acne with isolated lesions.
- *Kali brom 30*: Stressed teenagers.
- *Antimony crud 200*: Small, pointed lesions.
- *Causticum 200 alternating with Antimony crud 6*: Acne rosacea.
- *Hepar sulph 200:* Painful, pustular acne.

WARTS

[162]
Clinical presentation
Warts may be flat, horny, seborrheic, plantar or genital. While we know that warts are viral in origin (human papillomavirus or HPV), from a homeopathic viewpoint the miasmatic implications are more relevant. Genital or anal warts are contagious for susceptible individuals.

[163]
Differential diagnosis
Skin pigmentation lesions; skin cancers (check for undifferentiated edges); corns and calluses in plantar warts; some contagious skin diseases eg molluscum contagiosum.

[164]
Treatment
- *Antimony crud 6:* For common warts, without clear individualising symptoms. Given on alternate days for several months, this remedy will also cure many plantar warts.
- *Nitric ac 200:* Warts which occur at the muco-dermal junction (eg lips). Also for anal or genital warts occurring at the muco-dermal junction.
- *Thuja 200 alternating with Medorrhinum 200:* For genito-anal warts (not at the muco-dermal junction) prompt results can be seen by alternating these remedies.

LICHEN PLANUS

[165]
Clinical presentation
Lichen planus can occur either on the skin or in the mouth. The mouth lesions usually occur on the tongue, giving it a furry brown coating with bluish-white spots or lines. The skin lesions are itchy, flat, discreet, violet papules which may join into scaling patches. Sometimes the lesions have small, white lines. They are often found on the lower legs, with or without mouth lesions.

[166]
Differential diagnosis
Psoriasis (white-silvery scales but less itching); pityriasis rosea (oval, yellow to tan erythematous patches, with scaly edges and appearance similar to ringworm). Lichen sclerosis of the vagina causes some itching, but mostly soreness. In some cases this makes intercourse too painful. *Kreosotum 200,* repeated every 2nd day for weeks to months, is effective in many cases.

[167]
Treatment
- *Arsenicum 200 alternating with Antimony crud 6:* Lichen planus of the skin. Continue treatment for some months.
- *Hepar sulph 200:* Lichen planus of the mouth.
- *Kreosotum 200:* Lichen sclerosis of the vagina.

VITILIGO & LEUCODERMA

[168]
Clinical presentation
Absence of skin pigmentation, resulting in pale, white or discoloured patches.

Treatment
- *Mezereum 6:* This remedy gives the best results. Repeat the dose every second day for at least 18 months before choosing another remedy.
- *Bovista 200*: We have also found this remedy effective but its action is slower.
- *Arsenicum 200:* If the pigment disorder is pink or red.
- *Nitric ac 200:* Occurs at the muco-cutaneous junction.

ECZEMA & DERMATITIS

[169]
Overview
Clinical presentation
Differential Diagnosis
As with asthma, eczema and dermatitis may be intrinsic or extrinsic. In extrinsic or atopic conditions, the skin is inflamed and itchy. It may appear suddenly and spread quickly. Many skin diseases have no allergic or sensitivity background. These are classed as intrinsic.

Correct nutrition is essential in the management and treatment of any skin disease. Poor nutrition may be an impediment to cure.

Causations:
o *Food sensitivity*: More likely a contributing or sustaining factor in dermatitis. See the discussion of food sensitivity at [89] ff.
o *Food allergy*: An allergic reaction to a food substance will produce a rapid, itchy and inflamed eruption. See Allergy at [89] ff.
o *Allopathic medication*: Skin reactions can occur with many drugs, such as antibiotics or sulphur drugs.
o *Stress*: Sudden or prolonged stress can produce skin eruptions which improve once the stressful circumstances have passed.

[170]
Treatment
Skin problems are notoriously difficult to treat and can discourage any practitioner, whether they are a dermatologist or homeopath. However, homeopathy can offer spectacular results in obstinate cases.

The table on the following page is a general guide only. Miasmatic and constitutional treatment is often necessary to fully resolve the skin disease. The bowel nosodes, especially Morgan (Bach), are especially effective in children.

Keynotes in Eczema & Dermatitis

Location

Folds of skin (eg ears, groin, axilla)	*Graph 200*
Genitals	*Ars 200* *(Ars 200 alt Merc 200 for herpes; Merc 200 for balanitis)*
Lips	*Ars 200* *Merc 200* *Nit-ac 200 (muco-cutaneous junction)*
Muco-cutaneous junction	*Nit-ac 200*
Navel	*Ars 200*
Palms	*Petr 200 (cracking)*
Soles	*Sars 30 (cracking)*
Whole body	*Camph 200 (iatrogenic)* *Rhus-t 30 (non-iatrogenic)*

Presentation

Circumscribed	*Tub-b 200 (circles)* *Sep 200 (any shape)* *Tell 200 (intersecting circles)*
Cracking	*Petr 200* *Sars 30 (bleeding)*
Dryness and flaking	*Alumina 200*
Exfoliating	*Ars iod 200* *Kali-s 30* *Mez 200 (itching ichythiosis)* *Tub-b 200 (non-itching ichythiosis)*
Fungal	*Graph 200* *Sep 200 (ringworm – discrete rings)* *Tell 200 (ringworm – intersecting rings)*
Itching	*Mez 200 (main feature)*
Morbilliform	*Rhus t 30* *Puls 200*
Papular	*Ant-c 6*
Pink	*Ars 200*
Pustular	*Hep-s 200*
Red orifices	*Sulph 200* *Med 200 (nappy rash)*
Serous	*Graph 200*
Vesicular	*Rhus-t 30*

Children

Eczema, asthma & bowel disturbance	*Morg (Bach) 30*
Eczema & susceptibility to colds	*Calc 30*
Post-vaccination	*DTPa 30 (or respective vaccine)*

FEVER

Differential diagnosis
Finding the focus of infection when a patient has a fever is crucial but sometimes no cause can be found. Fevers caused by bacteria are higher than viral fevers. Physical examination is essential and may reveal:
o *Tonsillitis*
o *Chest infection*
o *Ear infection*
o *Tooth abcess*
o *Urinary tract infection (UTI)*
o *Pelvic inflammatory disease (PID)*
o *Viral infection eg influenza or childhood illness*
o *Meningitis.*

More obscure diagnoses may include:
o *Enteric fever*: Salmonella typhi and paratyphi, giardiasis, shigella. An early sign of enteric fever is gurgling sound in the caecum and drowsiness.
o *Acute pyelonephritis:* Following streptococcal infection: Fever with scanty urine, puffy face: the infection may have gone to kidneys.
o *Rheumatic fever*: Prior sore throat followed by joint pain and fever some weeks later.
o *Intestinal parasites*: Low chronic intermittent fever, weight loss, abdominal pain, possible itching of rectum and nose, nocturnal teeth grinding, insatiable or poor appetite.
o *Hepatitis*: Fever with nausea, jaundice and hepatomegaly.
o *Leukaemia*: Splenomegaly and prolonged intermittent fever.
o *Lymphoma:* Fever with lymphadenopathy and discrete glands.
o *Filliarosis:* Recurrent fever with non-pitting swelling of testes and feet (uncommon in the developed countries).

Treatment
The current trend of giving paracetamol to children when they have fevers is unnecessary. Fever is a natural symptom created by the body to fight infection. Fevers require no serious intervention unless they reach 39.5+.
The following remedies are useful for containing fever:

• *Ferrum phos 200:* The main remedy for fever up to 39.0.
• *Belladonna 200:* The main remedy for fever over 39.0 particularly if pupils are dilated or the patient is delirious.
• *Aconite 200:* High fever after cold wind exposure, particularly if the pupils are contracted and the patient is restless.
• *Gelsemium 6:* High fever with ptosis and dizziness.

In cases where all investigations produce no differential diagnosis and the patient appears well apart from ongoing fever:

- *Camphor 200:* The main remedy: two doses daily for up to one week where there are neither diagnosis nor individualising symptoms. *Camphor* is also effective in treating iatrogenic fever.
- *Tuberculinum bov 200:* One dose daily until there is a reaction where the fever is accompanied by nocturnal perspiration.
- *Arsenicum 200:* An intermittent fever appears at the same time each day.

VERTIGO

[172]
Clinical presentation
A sensation of spinning or other continuous movement in the head with nausea and loss of balance.

[173]
Differential diagnosis

1. Middle or inner ear pathology or functional disturbance must be investigated. Some examples are:
o Middle ear or eustachian catarrh
o Chronic otitis media
o Labyrinthitis
o Vestibular neuronitis
o Disturbances of the inner ear (8th cranial nerve).

2. Cervical spondylosis
3. Meniere's disease
4. Migraine
5. Pathology, eg, brain tumour, transient ischaemic attack, acoustic neuroma and neurological disorders
6. Anxiety.

[174]
Treatment
Where the cause of vertigo is unknown or the vertigo is unresponsive to treatment, refer for neurological assessment.
  The first two ear conditions listed above can be identified by inspection.
- *Pulsatilla 30 or 200* (with *Kali mur 3x* mixed): Middle ear or eustachian tube catarrh.
- *Conium 3 or Conium 3 mixed with Bryonia 30:* For **labyrinthitis**. If there is also tinnitus and loss of hearing, consider *Manganum* or *Sepia*.
- In **Meniere's disease** there is often nausea and vomiting with aggravation from every sound or least movement; impairment of hearing and tinnitus. The main remedies are *Bryonia, Theridion* and *Cuprum*.
- For vertigo of **migraine** where there is a rush of blood to the head: *Belladonna 200.* Also consider *Sanguinaria 200*.
- For vertigo associated with **cervical spondylosis** or other neck pathology, *Conium 3* is also often effective. If *Conium* fails, then *Cimicifuga 30* should next be given regularly for several weeks. Also consider referral for osteopathy.
Treatment for chronic otitis media can be found at [14].

MUSCULOSKELETAL

OSGOOD SCHLATTER'S DISEASE

[175]
Clinical presentation
Swelling and tenderness of the tibial tuberosity. X-ray may show irregular ossification of the tibial tubercle. Most common in teenage males.

[176]
Treatment
- *Ledum 200:* Most cases respond slowly to repeated doses.
- *Calcarea carb 200:* Consider alternating with *Ledum*, since this will assist overall bone metabolism and development.

ARTHRITIS

[177]
Clinical presentation
o *Osteoarthritis*: stiffness after rest, pain worse on joint movement and loss of joint function. Local tenderness, occasional slight swelling. Common in middle age onwards or after injury.
o *Rheumatoid arthritis*: severe and progressive joint pain with inflammation and eventually deformity. Generally occurs in patients before the age of 40.

[178]
Differential diagnosis
Psoriatic arthritis; Reiter's syndrome; gout; rheumatic fever; Ross River Fever (and other viral pathogens); systemic lupus erythematosus; Lyme disease; septic arthritis (eg gonococcal).

[179]
Treatment
Treatment of rheumatoid arthritis is complex and difficult, especially in advanced pathology. Since rheumatoid arthritis is an autoimmune disease, correct nutrition is paramount. Allergic triggers are a factor in some cases. A history of viral infections (particularly if they preceded onset) is relevant.

A diet rich in omega-3 fatty acids, low in red meat and exclusion of food allergens or sensitivities are vital for effective management of arthritis. Glucosamine and chondroitin sulphate can assist in cartilage repair and omega-3 oils reduce inflammation (provided there is no sensitivity or allergy to them) and are thus of value in the treatment of both types of arthritis.

- *Cimicifuga 30:* In simple osteoarthritis of the hands and cervical spondylosis, with no other individualising symptoms, *Cimicifuga* achieves results if repeated every second day for months. It has an affinity for the joints of the fingers and neck. *Cimicifuga* works equally well in males and females.
- *Kalmia 6:* Also used in treatment of arthritis of the small joints, but there is deformity of the joints as well as pain and inflammation.
- *Ledum 200:* In osteoarthritis of the knee, *Ledum* should be tried first when there is swelling present.
- *Symphytum 200*: Where there is a clear history of trauma to the joint, start with *Symphytum* 200, repeated often for a least one month. In osteoarthritis of large joints, eg the hip, knee and shoulder, alternate *Symphytum 200* with *Calcarea phos 3x trit. Calcarea phos* has the ability to rebuild cartilage.
- *Rheumatoid arthritis nosode 30*: Rheumatoid arthritis is a difficult disease. We have experienced some success with this nosode, alternating with either *Cimicifuga* or *Kalmia*, as described above.
- *Salicylic ac 200*: Arthritis in post-menopausal women.

GOUT

[180]
Clinical presentation
Severe pain of one or more peripheral joints caused by monosodium urate crystal deposits in the joints. The most common joint affected is the first metatarsophalangeal joint of the great toe.

[181]
Differential diagnosis
Acute inflammatory arthritis (eg gonococcal or pneumococcal) or rheumatoid arthritis.

[182]
Treatment
- *Colchicum 30:* The main medicine for acute gout. Repeat for many months for recurrent gout.
- *Benzoic ac 200:* For chronic gout with formation of crystalline nodes in multiple joints. There may be a concomitant symptom of strong smelling urine.
- *Cimicifuga 30:* useful in some cases of gout which affects multiple small joints, however inflammation is mild.

A low purine diet and supplements which alkalise the tissues such as celery seed are recommended. Also check the allopathic medications of the patient: drugs such as the thiazide diuretics can increase uric acid.

ANXIETY

[183]
Clinical presentation
Everyone suffers anxiety at times. Unexplained anxiety, or anxiety out of proportion to the triggering events, can be treated with homeopathy. Unresolved emotional issues or difficulty in relationships should be referred for counselling or psychotherapy. A well-chosen remedy can help this process.

Symptoms of anxiety include: panic attacks, fainting, poor sleep, and difficult concentration.

[184]
Differential diagnosis
Hyper- (or sometimes hypo-) thyroidism (including Grave's disease). Side effects of some medications. Over-use of stimulants (eg caffeine or recreational drugs). Hypoglycaemia (anxiety worse after sugar or missing meals). Pituitary tumour. Tachycardia. Hormonal imbalances. Oestrogen or progesterone dominance. A fine tremor of the hands may suggest one of the above.

[185]
Treatment
The correctly chosen remedy does wonders for patients with anxiety. Most remedies would normally be given in higher potencies: at least the 200th, and repeated as needed. If higher, such as giving *Opium* for fear of a specific fright, we may give one dose of 10M or 50M. Be sure to look for the underlying causes of anxiety and treat accordingly.

Here are some common prescriptions.

- *Opium:* There is a clear event in the past which, when brought to mind, creates anxiety in the present. The repertory describes this as 'fear of the fright'. Opium is specific for this type of fear.
- *Gelsemium:* Anxiety is associated with dizziness; feels as though going to pass out. There may be a sensation of weight or thickness in the head. Thinking is heavy or cloudy. Palpitations or tremor occurs before ordeals.
- *Moschus:* Anxiety is focused in the chest, with a sense of suffocation, dyspnoea and chest pain. It has the '*Aconite*' fear of imminent death.
- *Ignatia:* Hysteric symptoms with tightness around the throat, needing to take a deep breath. Anxiety is somaticised, often felt in the throat or abdomen.
- *Argentum nit:* This remedy is effective where there is unequivocal claustrophobia: eg s/he absolutely cannot go into a tunnel at all without suffering extreme anxiety.
- *Folliculinum 30:* Unexplained anxiety as a side-effect from taking the oral contraceptive pill or HRT: see Oestrogen Dominance at [56]. The pill should be discontinued and the patient given *Folliculinum 30* every second day for several weeks.

- *Calcarea carb*: Anxiety stems from a perception of one being intellectually inferior or not up to the task. She feels she is stupid, and cannot follow simple instructions. Easily intimidated by those she perceives as more intelligent than herself.
- *Silicea*: Whilst similar to *Calcarea carb*, *Silicea's* sense of self is very fragile. Anything perceived as criticising or threatening to his sense of who he is creates tremendous anxiety. He will defer to others so this fragility is not put to the test.
- *Lycopodium*: Anxiety from a self-perception of weakness or incapacity which will result in others thinking less of him, or laughing at him. He will maintain every effort to put on a solid and capable *persona*, yet underneath he is an insecure mess. He has poor confidence when in public yet is bullying or irritable in the safety of his home environment.
- *Stramonium*: Terror with a history of fear of being alone in the dark: must have the light on.
- *Phosphorus*: Oversensitive and impressionable. For example to: psychic phenomena, visual impressions (cannot watch horror films), other people's emotions, storms, dark. May have a history of sleepwalking.

For 'anxiety' which has one of the causes listed in Differential Diagnosis, above, the remedy must address the underlying cause.

For example:
- o 'Anxiety' experienced as a result of Grave's disease should be given *Iodum 200*: see Hyperthyroidism at [190].
- o A woman suffering anxiety who takes the oral contraceptive pill and has oestrogen dominance must discontinue the pill and may require *Folliculinum 30*. See [56].

HYPOTHYROIDISM (MYXOEDEMA)

[186]
Clinical presentation
When a patient presents with fatigue, weight gain and hair loss, include hypothyroidism in the diagnostic possibilities. Not every case of hypothyroidism will have an elevated TSH: in some cases the free T4 needs to be measured to verify underactivity. Free T4 is not usually measured unless especially requested, so vigilance is needed. A goitre may be palpable.
 Common hypothyroid symptoms:

General
o Generalised body ache or paresthesia
o Sensation of a lump in the throat
o Dizziness
o Breathlessness
o Fatigue, weakness and poor concentration
o Progressive weight gain
o Goitre.

Female
o History of menorrhagia, amenorrhoea or irregularity
o Sighing.

GIT
o Constipation
o Abdominal distension.

Face
o Smooth, puffy and expressionless face of myxoedema
o Dull expression
o Malar flush
o Hair loss (including outer half of eyebrows).

Skin
o Cold, dry hands and thickened skin
o Cracking dermatitis (rhagades).

Cardiovascular
o Hypotension
o Palpitations or slow pulse
o Angina.

[187]
Differential diagnosis
Oestrogen dominance (including side effects from the oral contraceptive pill) or other hormonal irregularities, eg Polycystic Ovarian Syndrome, hursutism. Iatrogenic disease (eg long term use of corticosteroids). Amenorrhoea from non-thyroid causes. Other endocrine diseases.

[188]
Treatment
It is more common for a patient to present for homeopathy in the early stages of under-active thyroid, when their TSH is within normal range. Here, patients complain of excessive tiredness, weight changes and hair loss or cracked nails. These patients respond well to:

• *Thyroidinum 200*: Repeat every second day for many weeks.

• *Ignatia 200:* Anxiety, with disturbed sleep and possibly a sensation of lump in the throat.

• *Gelsemium 200:* Fatigue and excessive weakness. Hypothyroid patients who have amenorrhoea respond well to this remedy, with a restoration of the menses soon occurring.

• *Calcarea carb 200:* Where obesity is the only true symptom, *Calcarea carb* can be alternated with *Thyroidinum.*

[189]
Summary
• *Thyroidinum 200*: The main remedy.
• *Ignatia 200*: Disturbed sleep, anxiety, lump in throat.
• *Gelsemium 200*: Extreme fatigue, dizziness, possibly amenorrhoea.
• *Calcarea Carb 200*: Obesity.

HYPERTHYROIDISM (THYROTOXICOSIS)

[190]
Clinical presentation
Sudden unexplained anxiety, hyperactivity, insomnia, palpitations, fatigue or weight loss. Goitre may be palpable. The most common cause of hyperthyroidism is Grave's disease, an autoimmune disease in which there are antibodies against the thyroid TSH receptor.
Common symptoms are:

General
o   Goitre
o   Increased appetite
o   Weight loss
o   Gradual weakness
o   Excessive sweating
o   Insomnia
o   Nervousness or restlessness
o   Tremor
o   Heat intolerance.

Appearance
o   Fixed stare
o   Exophthalmos
o   Upper eyelid retraction.

Cardiovascular
o   Tachycardia (during sleep differentiates other causes)
o   Finger clubbing in myxoedema
o   Forceful apex beat, basal crepitation or atrial fibrillation.

Urinary
o   Glycosuria.

[191]
Differential diagnosis
Anxiety, diabetes, malignancy.

[192]
Treatment
• *Iodum 200*: The main remedy, which should be repeated initially every second day.
Iodum is effective in many cases, including Grave's disease. All the typical features are in this remedy:
o   Feeling of or actual protrusion of the eyes with twitching of the lids
o   Tachycardia

- o Aggravation from the least exertion with fainting
- o Excessive irritability, restlessness
- o Debility with weakness and dyspnoea on ascending
- o Excessive perspiration and intolerance of heat
- o Voracious appetite with weight loss; there is hunger intolerance: s/he must eat every few hours.

Iodum can restore normal thyroid function, avoiding the need for allopathic medication. The response can be rapid, provided the remedy is repeated every second day to begin with. *Iodum* can also be used in *unstable* hyperthyroidism, where allopathic medication is already being taken but is not adequately managing symptoms.

While it is advisable that regular pathology reports are requested throughout treatment, the patient's symptoms (or absence of them) offer the best marker for homeopathic assessment of progress.

RAYNAUD'S DISEASE/PHENOMENON

[193]
Clinical presentation
Intermittent attacks of cyanosis of the fingers or toes, with coldness. In milder cases, there is pallor, or redness. In advanced cases, the skin tears and infection follows. If the disease is idiopathic it is called Raynaud's disease, or if it is secondary to pathology, such as scleroderma, it is called Raynaud's phenomenon. Attacks can be triggered by emotional upset.

[194]
Treatment
- *Secale 6 or 30:* The main remedy. The lower potencies are preferable, and should be repeated often. It may not *cure* Raynaud's, but the patient can become symptom-free relatively quickly.
- *Arsenicum 200 or Lachesis 200:* For infection in the fingertips.
- *Lachesis 200*: The preferred remedy for infection if there is blue/black colour or burning sensation (compare *Anthracinum*).
- *Hepar sulph 6:* Where Raynaud's is secondary to scleroderma, and the scleroderma infiltrates the oesophagus, *Hepar sulph 6* affords much relief from the reflux and constriction.

[195]
Summary
- *Secale 6 or 30*: The main remedy.
- *Arsenicum 200*: Infection in the fingertips.
- *Lachesis 200:* Infection with blue/black colour.
- *Hepar sulph 6*: Pyloric or oesophageal problems associated with scleroderma.

DIABETES

Clinical presentation
Excessive thirst, hunger, nocturnal urination, and weight loss, are primary symptoms of a blood sugar disorder.

Type I, or 'juvenile' diabetes, is always insulin dependent and there is no conventional cure. Patients with Type I do not usually seek homeopathic treatment for their diabetes; they may do so for associated symptoms.

Type II diabetes used to be called 'maturity onset', as it only occurred in middle aged people. The name was changed to 'Type II' due to the increasing incidence in young people. Type II is diet and lifestyle related. Type II patients are more likely to seek a homeopathic solution *before* the need arises to start insulin. These patients will have been placed on a sugar-free diet, and may be taking an oral hypoglycaemic.

Well managed diabetics may still develop diabetic sequelae, even though their blood sugar is stable. Some patients do not respond well to insulin, and their blood sugar remains unstable despite the best allopathic interventions.

As the disease becomes firmly established, other symptoms are possible:
- Peripheral neuropathy: tingling, numbness, burning, sensation of walking on air
- Glycosuria
- Weight loss
- Retinopathy causing hazy vision due to diabetic cataract or papilloedema
- Fungal infections
- Boils
- Diabetic ulcer
- Peripheral skin infections.

[197]
Differential diagnosis
Polyuria: UTI, prostatic hypertrophy. Other endocrine disorders eg hyper/hypothyroidism. Other (non-diabetic) neuropathies. If local ischaemia: Raynaud's phenomenon; ischaemia from other causes: eg atherosclerosis.

[198]
Treatment
A diet with a low glycaemic index and a supplement of the glucose tolerance factor chromium are recommended. Vitamin E 500-1000iu daily and 100mg Co-Enzyme Q10 are recommended for cardiovascular support.

- *Helonias 200:* Blood sugar fluctuations can be kept more stable, and overall blood sugar will slowly decrease, with *Helonias*. This is repeated every second day, then reduced by one day for each month of treatment, provided the patient is stable. This protocol takes at least 12 months. The remedy works better in pre-insulin dependent diabetes. If the remedy is not working, alternate with *Lycopodium 200.*

- *Hypericum 200:* We have also treated diabetic neuropathy where the patient has developed symptoms while under allopathic care. We have found *Hypericum 200* effective in neuropathy, provided it is repeated regularly for at least one month.
- *Arsenicum 200:* Where the neuropathy has severe, stabbing pain (neuritis), alternate *Hypericum* with *Arsenicum 200.*
- *Secale 6 or 30:* If *Arsenicum* fails for neuropathy, *Secale* may be effective if there is peripheral ischaemia.
- *Zincum 200:* Chorea, twitching of muscles and weakness of the extremities.

[199]
Summary
- *Helonias 200*: The main remedy.
- *Hypericum 200*: Diabetic neuropathy.
- *Arsenicum 200*: Acute neuritis.
- *Secale 6 or 30*: Neuritis with ischaemia.
- Zincum 200: Chorea, twitching, weakness.

DISEASES OF THE EYE

PTERYGIUM

[200]
Clinical presentation
Pterygium is a fleshy growth of bulbar conjunctiva on the cornea. Symptoms may be stigmatism, or local irritation. It is classed as a benign neoplasm.

[201]
Differential diagnosis
Glaucoma (pain +++ and greater vision disturbance); iritis (pain ++ with photophobia); cataract (progressive, painless loss of vision).

[202]
Treatment
As with any pathology, remedies take time to produce results. We have successfully treated pterygium with *Mercurius sol 1M*, repeated once weekly: treatment time was eight months.

CONJUNCTIVITIS

[203]
Clinical presentation
Inflammation, pain of the conjunctiva, photophobia, watery or purulent discharge. Agglutination if there is purulence.

[204]
Differential diagnosis
Blepharitis: inflammation of the margins of the eyelids (For blepharitis *Argentum met 200* works better than the remedies for conjunctivitis.)

[205]
Treatment
Many practitioners routinely give *Euphrasia* in the treatment of conjunctivitis, but this remedy only has a small scope. *Euphrasia* is effective for a non-purulent, watery discharge, which is a less common feature in conjunctivitis. Most cases present with a muco-purulent, yellow discharge, which causes the eyelids to stick together after sleeping (agglutination). These symptoms respond to:
• *Argentum nit 200*: The main remedy for purulence and agglutination. (The patient does not have to have anxiety in enclosed spaces for this remedy to be effective.)
• *Belladonna 3*: This remedy is sometimes needed if there is acute inflammation of the conjunctiva with severe photophobia.
• *Euphrasia 200*: Non-purulent, watery discharge.

[206]
Summary
• *Argentum nit 200*: The main remedy: agglutination and purulence.
• *Belladonna 3*: Acute inflammation with photophobia.
• *Euphrasia 200:* Watery discharge.

MOUTH ULCERS

[207]
Clinical presentation
Circumscribed ulcer on the buccal mucosa with pinpoint pain.

[208]
Differential diagnosis
Any persistent ulcer which does not heal within approximately one week may be malignant. Leucoplakia is a pre-cancerous condition which generally occurs in adults. Apthae (white spots in thrush) or vesicles (eg foot and mouth disease).

[209]
Treatment
- *Mercurius sol 200:* The main remedy.
- *Nitric ac 200:* Exceptionally sharp pain, or lesions occur at the muco-cutaneous junction, ie corners of the mouth.
- *Borax 30:* A superficial ulcer with rawness rather than sharp pain, more likely to occur in children.

PART 4: ILLNESSES OF MEN

BENIGN PROSTATIC HYPERTROPHY (BHP)

[210]
Clinical presentation
Frequent urination; feeble stream; dribbling at close of urination; occasionally pain at the close of urination (if there is prostatitis).

[211]
Differential diagnosis
Malignancy of the prostate; bladder infection (uncommon in men unless paraplegic); diabetes.

[212]
Treatment
Patients should be encouraged to adopt dietary factors beneficial for prostate health. Foods high in zinc and omega 3 fatty acids should be encouraged. All legumes and seeds contain beneficial micronutrients for prostate health. Avoid foods which have a diuretic action, such as coffee and tea, especially in the evening, so that sleep is not disturbed by frequent urging for urination.

The best remedy for the above symptoms is:

• *Sarsaparilla 30. Sarsaparilla* can also be used for acute prostatitis and bladder infection, if there is pain at the close of urination. In hypertrophy it should be repeated regularly for many months.

• *Medorrhinum 200:* If there is a history of sexually transmitted disease, *Medorrhinum* may be more effective.

• *Thuja 30:* Alternate with *Sarsaparilla* if hypertrophy is increasing even though the *symptoms* have improved on *Sarsaparilla.*

• *Conium 3:* Has a therapeutic reputation for tumours of the prostate. It is more effective for hard tumours.

• *Clematis 30:* Use this remedy when there is interrupted flow, or urine only passes in tiny drips.

PART 5
Case Examples in the Treatment of Chronic Disease

These case examples illustrate the need for flexible prescribing approaches in practice.

Case 1: Sam, male, age 4 – Gut and Behavioural Disturbance in Child
This case illustrates the need for aetiological prescribing before the constitutional medicine is given. We could not give the constitutional medicine initially because:
1. *Other symptoms obscured the required constitutional remedy.*
2. *This is a clear case of iatrogenically induced disease, or 'never well since'. This layer of the disease phenomenon needed priority treatment.*

Symptoms:

Head banging.
Smelly diarrhoea and abdominal pain.
Unexplained temper tantrums: does not wish to be touched or even looked at. Suddenly yells at strangers. Pretends he's a dog and growls at people.
Speech delay; writing delay.
Hates being touched, especially on the head.
Does not like to make eye contact.
Ongoing undiagnosed headaches and abdominal pains.
Irritable, cross, resists attempts by parents for affection.
Hypersensitivity reactions to many foods.
Poor appetite.
Night terrors.

At the first visit he was already taking Neocate and Metameal. He had been placed on formula at birth, since his older brother had had anaphylactic reactions to many foods. He received surgery for pyloric stenosis. At 10 months he contracted a severe case of salmonella infection and was hospitalised with diarrhoea. At 11 months there were recurring ear infections. Antibiotics were given and grommets inserted. His hearing became *worse* and he *stopped talking*.

Family History: Mother: allergies. Mother's father: alcoholism and violence.
Sam's mother has a history of adult onset allergies. She has anaphylactic reactions to nuts.

Many of these symptoms present in children diagnosed with ADHD. When we see strong symptoms of speech delay, refusal to make eye contact and dislike for being touched, varying degrees of autistic spectrum disorder may be diagnosed. Neither of these medical diagnoses is particularly helpful in our experience. What is helpful is discovering the causative factors in each individual case, and treating those factors. Many children placed in either of the two above categories, have a variety of different aetiologies which are white-washed by placing them into a 'disorder' box.
Sam had not yet been diagnosed with either of the above disorders. Although one could imagine that if his symptom picture failed to improve, this would be the diagnostic outcome as he grew older.

When Sam first attended for treatment he displayed symptoms we typically see in children who have gut-brain disorders.

We know that the gut is full of neuro-transmitters. In fact, one could regard the gut wall as an extension of the brain itself. Many children in the Western world today have this problem. They experience behavioural reactions after eating certain foods. Even children who do not fall into the 'gut-brain' spectrum of disorders still react to some foods: just feed your child colourings and preservatives all day and see what their behaviour is like by dinner time!

In children like Sam, we know that the gut wall is hyper-responsive to certain food stimuli. The gut wall has become too permeable, so that partially digested food substances which normally do not pass through into the blood stream are now passing through. The neuro-transmitters in the gut wall also have faulty recognition systems. They classify normally harmless food proteins as antagonists. This sends messages to the brain that the body is being attacked. Then the child experiences sensitivity reactions, such as abdominal pain, bloating, inflammation of the bowel wall, mood changes, disordered bowel function. In severe cases, as with nut allergy, we get anaphylactic reactions.

Our treatment of Sam began with ridding his intestinal system of what we considered were the possibility of ongoing parasitic infections. Night terrors, abdominal pain and irritability are strong markers for parasitic infection. His dislike of being touched or looked at led us to begin treatment with a course of *Cina 200*: one dose every second day. During the next two weeks he passed tiny black spots in his stools. His stools began to become properly formed, his smelly flatulence improved, his appetite and abdominal pain improved slightly. His night terrors improved. Despite these encouraging signs, there were minimal changes to his overall behavioural problems. He also continued to experience abdominal pain and headaches. So we followed with a one month course of *Nux vom 30* alternating with *Stannum 200*. Again we saw further improvement: fewer night terrors, less abdominal pain and flatulence. Yet he still complained of infrequent headaches and abdominal pain. Clearly, we needed to take a 'layered' approach to treatment.

We suspect vaccinosis when we see groupings of symptoms like these:
o Frequent waking
o Nocturnal fevers
o Repeated otitis media &/or middle ear effusion.
o Repeated coughs, colds, wheezes, unexplained by circumstances or family history
o Weight loss or poor appetite
o Aggravation from vaccination
o Symptoms began shortly after vaccination
o Head-banging.

Persistent head banging, without any evidence of middle ear infection, should be viewed as a sign of cerebral irritation, and is often a strong pointer to vaccinosis.

We next prescribed for Sam a course of the homeopathic potency of the *DPT/Pedvax* vaccination in the manner described by Dr Tinus Smits, with daily repeated doses of 30, then 200 and finally 1M (10 to 14 days of each potency in ascending order, with a short consultation between each to assess results). *This vaccination, normally given to babies at two, four and six months of age, is in our experience, the one which most commonly produces long term sequelae. Even though the MMR vaccine has been in the spotlight recently as a possible causative factor in autistic spectrum disorder, in our experience the DPT (or DTPa) is more often a major factor. However, DPT (DTPa) is more likely to cause functional disturbances, such as to gut or ear, nose and throat).*

Sam's response to this prescription was incredible. One day he was an angry child who refused all affection. The next day he went to his mother and said for the first time: "I love you Mummy". Over the next few weeks his speech development rocketed. His unexplained tantrums improved. The head banging stopped. His appetite improved. His bowel function completely returned to normal (having previously been improved by the *Cina, Nux and Stannum*). (There were clear responses to the *DPT/Pedvax* 30th and 200th, but nothing was noticed with the 1M.)

Rationale for prescription:
If you look at Sam in a layered approach, this is how we think his health was affected:

1. Mother had strong tendency to food allergy (with anaphylaxis). Possibly there are other genetic factors considering the mother's father.
2. Sam is born with this inherited tendency.
3. Sam is inappropriately given the usual vaccinations. He reacts to one or more of the vaccines: either the viral components, the animal cells upon which the vaccine was cultured, or other components in the vaccine.
4. He contracts 'salmonella' (or is this his body's response to a vaccination, or a sign that he is not able to handle many normal foods?)
5. He has ongoing health problems affecting his intestinal and nervous systems.

Treatment was to peel off these disease layers in *reverse* order:
1. Remove any intestinal pathogens
2. Antidote presumed side effects of vaccination
3. Constitutional or miasmatic prescription to reduce allergic and hypersensitive tendencies.

We next gave Sam a single dose of *Tuberculinum bov 10M*, which provoked a high fever and sore throat. His writing skills began to develop and his tantrums were better. However, he could still be violent with his brothers (biting, punching). Now that so much of his disease pathology had been 'peeled off', we had the opportunity to observe his behaviour more clearly. These violent outbursts tended to occur whenever any attention was given to his brothers. In other words, he was jealous. There is a great little rubric in Peter Tumminello's repertory, *The Child's Mind and Behaviour*: "Jealously, baby, when a new, takes the attention of the family away".

We also find the rubric "Jealousy, rage, with" in Murphy's *Repertory* with only one remedy.

Our next prescription was therefore *Hyoscyamus 1M*, one dose. Since this remedy, Sam's behaviour has been excellent, with far fewer tantrums. His speech and writing are now excellent, with clear enunciation of his words.

In cases like Sam's, where we see a clinically indisputable result, this confirms the view that the DPT/Pedvax vaccination is likely to have been a causative factor in the disease, otherwise an antidote to that vaccine is unlikely to have had any effect. While a majority of children pass through the vaccination schedule without long term side effects, there is a minority who do not. Certainly, in children with a strong family history of allergy or food sensitivity, the need for vaccination needs to be carefully reviewed.

Case 2: GB, male, age 29 – Asthma and Sinusitis

This case illustrates what every homeopath dreads: there is a paucity of individualising symptoms. In this case, we need to use a keynote approach, or give what we have described as the 'main medicine' to treat this disease. We would continue with this medicine while improvement is experienced, only changing if improvement stops and/or a new symptom picture forms.

Symptoms:

Asthma with itchy eyes, nose and throat. Runny nose. Wheeze.
Rhinitis/hayfever.
Fatigue.
Began as a child, with absence of symptoms through teens, now returned.
Aggravation: wind and summer.

Family History
Father: rheumatoid arthritis; multiple allergies.

Medications
Ventolin. Becotide. Antihistamines.

Analysis
This is a one-sided case with no individualising symptoms. Prescription is only possible on keynote symptoms, or 'main remedy' style.

Prescription: *Arsenicum 6 twice daily.*
Avoid yeast.

First follow up: three weeks
Asthma > by 25-50%
Itchy eyes > 50%
Itchy nose & throat > 50%.

No Becotide or Antihistamines used. Some use of Ventolin.

Skin has improved (dry scaly patches – not mentioned in first visit).

Itching has reduced when he exercises (not mentioned in first visit).

Second follow up: two months
Sinus and asthma flare ups persist, but are of less severity and duration lasting only half hour.
Aggravation: dust, dog hair.
Using Ventolin a little more, the *Arsenicum* not now working as well. But still using Ventolin only half as much compared to before starting treatment.
Itchy skin, especially after eating white bread.

No Becotide or anti-histamines used.

Mucus on chest is persistent, but now mostly clear. (Not mentioned in previous visits).

Prescription: *Arsenicum 6 once daily; Tuberculinum bov 200 once weekly.*

Third follow up: four months
After taking *Tuberculinum*, he experienced six days of sinus pain, which did not go to the chest (normally sinus infections go to the chest).

After the second dose of *Tuberculinum*, some itching and running nose, but no other reactions.

Recent nose block (from the spring wattles).

Some wheezing: using ventolin approximately four times daily, as before.

New Prescription: *Kali carb 200: One dose every second day.*

Fourth follow up: seven months
"Fantastic".

No symptoms apart from slight wheezing. Using ventolin only once per day.

Goes out without taking his ventolin ("I never used to do this").

The patient is instructed on further doses, then discharged.

Rationale for prescriptions given:
o *Arsenicum* we have described under Asthma in the asthma mix as a reliever of acute asthma. We have also described *Arsenicum* under Sinusitis & Rhinitis: it has itching, bland coryza and wheezing. It is thus a reliable remedy for commencing treatment since it covers all the particulars of the case.
o *Tuberculinum Bov*: we have described under Asthma as a reliable medicine when there is a clear allergic diathesis where there are multiple allergies.
o *Kali carb* is also described under Asthma: it is the main remedy to use where there are no clear symptoms for another remedy.

We may well have given *Kali carb* at the first visit and achieved a more rapid result. However, *Arsenicum* was chosen because the case also had a strong emphasis on hay fever with itching eyes and nose.

Case 3: LL, female, age 35 – Asthma and Sinusitis

This case illustrates a clinical situation where one can rely on the mentals to sustain one's remedy choice. In this case there is an **observable, direct relationship** *between the patient's mentals and the manifestation of physical symptoms.*

Symptoms:
o Asthma since age 6.

Aggravation: after catching colds; mango (+ hives), crustaceans, some Thai food; cigarette smoke+++; dust; dog hair; exercise; before menses; winds.

Chronic mouth breather without nasal discharge.

History
Tonsil- & adenoidectomy at 8 years old due to history of tonsillitis.
Eye infections, styes, cysts.
Shingles twice.
Glandular fever (asymptomatic)
Car accident at 17yrs with long term thoracic pain.

Particulars
Cracked heels.
Throat infections +++.
Deviated septum.
Rhinitis.

Mentals
Perfectionist
Works in drug and alcohol.
"Lack of values and loyalty in people these days".
Developed mouth ulcers and cold sores the day after the September 11 bombings.
Vivid dreams: always thinking about something.
Social justice very important.

Family History
Father: polyps, Irritable Bowel Syndrome.

Medications
Flixotide twice weekly. Ventolin two puffs once daily.

Prescription: *Causticum 200: One dose every second day. Arsenicum 6 as needed.*

Follow up: Five weeks later
Symptoms aggravated first two to three weeks. Now improved.
Currently using NO flixotide or ventolin. "I'm never without my drugs".

Arsenicum 6 is used as needed with good effect.
A little rhinitis, but not much.
Able to breathe through her nose.

Prescription: *Continue Causticum 200 every third day; Arsenicum 6 as needed.*

Rationale for prescription:
There is a *clear, direct and observable relationship* between mentals and the arising of physical symptoms. This patient's sympathetic response to the 9/11 bombings produced a physical pathology (cold sores). This remedy choice is supported by symptoms such as aggravation from winds; preoccupation with social justice; tendency to herpetic eruptions; tendency to laryngitis. *A clear relationship between mental states and physical symptoms must be observed before relying on a 'mentals' prescription.*

Case 4: KH, female, age 26 – Asthma and Sinusitis
This case illustrates the reliance one can place on a clear and strong modality. The modality in this case is the most important prescribing symptom and all other symptoms are subservient to it.

Symptoms:
Asthma, sinusitis, allergies.
Main allergic triggers: dairy, yeast, green apples (aggravate wheezing); sugar (causes palpitations), vinegar (aggravates wheezing), cats+++ (aggravates hives).
Post-nasal drip with thick mucus and pain at forehead.
Nose block after consuming trigger foods.
Middle ear fluid and sensation of fullness.
Eczema in humid weather.
Aggravation of symptoms: humid weather+++; wind; night.
Amelioration of symptoms: dry climate (no asthma for six months while in Jindabyne which is a dry climate. Symptoms aggravated when she moved to a humid climate.)

Other symptoms
Occipital headaches during sleep.
Sleep very restless.
Migraines left side with aura, ever since having a caesarian section.
Periods are heavy, irregular, with black clots and much blood.
Produced too much milk during breast feeding.
Vaginal thrush from recent antibiotics.
Thoracic pain since caesarian section.

History
Severe eczema with much use of topical cortisone.
Frequent colds, tonsillitis, bronchitis, pneumonia twice.
Surgery twice for nasal polyps.
Chicken pox: bronchitis and other complications followed.

Mentals
Feels distanced or removed from others.
Depression after friends have moved away from her area. Feels isolated after having moved to her new location.
Grief – feels she has lost her spiritual/healing ability. Sees beings out of her peripheral vision.
Hopelessness.
Anger: partner's family not listening to her re raising her children. No respect from his family. Holds back anger and withdraws. Feels like throwing herself under a car.
Cravings: coffee, tea, red wine. No addictive tendencies.

Dreams
Being chased by murderers.
Falling.
Being stabbed.
Her children drowning.

Family History
Father: asthma, prostate cancer.
Mother: cervical cancer, Hashimoto's thyroiditis, back pain.
Brother: mild asthma.
Mother's brother: asthma.
Mother's mother: pancreatic & liver cancer.

Previous remedies given (potencies unknown)
Ignatia: provoked suicidal thoughts.
Thuja: aggravated thrush and physical symptoms without improvement.
Medorrhinum: aggravated nightmares, felt more withdrawn but also more stable.
Staphysagria: no effect.

Prescription: Natrum sulph 30: One dose every second day.

Follow up: Three weeks later
No asthma.
Only slight sinusitis with southerly change.
Sleeping much better: previously was waking every few hours.
No migraines.
No nose block.
Ears not blocked but some "ringing". (Old symptom return)
Some eczema on fingers but not itchy. Eczema slightly aggravated.
Periods returned next day after starting remedy, with normal bleeding and no pain.
Craving for coffee, red wine is gone. Now wants chicken.
Dumped on by her partner's family over how she raises her children. This time her partner supported here (in the past he has not).
"I felt stronger – she [mother-in-law] didn't affect me so much".
Cried in front of my own mother ("I usually never show tears to anyone").
Feels quiet and still inside – not depressed ("depression is my normal response").
Vivid dreams of body parts.

Analysis: Simillimum found due to symptoms improving on many levels.

Treatment: Continue at same dose.

***Rationale for prescription*:**
- Most important symptom: illness is aggravated by humid weather. Other symptoms which support the prescription:
- The sycotic miasm is evident in the aggravation from humidity and the history of polyps.
- Her feelings of separateness, withdrawal, grief and depression support consideration of one of the *Natrums*.

Case 5: NB:, female, age 5 - Middle Ear Effusion

This case illustrates the importance of choosing a remedy which is capable of resolving a middle ear effusion. An effusion, using our definition in the introduction, is a pathology, since the disease outcome is a long-standing change to the physical structure of tissues (effusion plus tympanum bulge and reduced motility). The remedy chosen is the 'main remedy' indicated for middle ear effusion, even though one could choose other remedies based on the generals of the case. The particulars in this case have been considered more important than the generals. This approach, though contrary to usual homeopathic thought, may be necessary in cases involving a physical pathology.

Symptoms:

Reduced hearing: cannot hear unless she turns her ear towards the speaker. Asks for the television to be turned up. Speaks loudly. Pronunciation is poor.
While generally described as easy going, she may also be stubborn+++ or 'emotional'.
Fears: the wind at night; the dark.
Sleep: restless, may wake twice during the night.
Desires: fruit, sweets, raw carrot, cheese.
Averse: vegetables, orange juice.
Thirsty: drinks up to 2 litres per day.

Family History
Mother: eczema.
Sister: dairy sensitivity.

History
Born prematurely.
Six ear infections as a toddler.

Examination
Ear drums show poor translucence, dark colour, no light reflexes. The tympanogram shows poor motility.

Prescription: *Pulsatilla 30: One dose every second day. Exclude dairy products from the diet.*

At her second visit hearing was normal. On examination her drums were normal.

Rationale for prescription:
One might consider remedies such as *Calcarea carb*, *Silicea* or *Tuberculinum* (stubbornness, fear of dark and diseases of middle ear) and these remedies *may* have had a beneficial effect. However, *Pulsatilla* has been chosen *despite the*

generals of the case because *Pulsatilla* is the main remedy for resolving middle ear effusion. In this case, the action of the remedy was rapid and effective.

We would normally advise restoration of dairy in the diet once the child is well, to see if she can then tolerate dairy or not. This was recommended and this case and no further ear problems occurred.

The following case takes this idea further.

Case 6: AV, male, age 40- Chronic Otitis Externa

This case combines two approaches. First, remedies based entirely on the pathology are chosen (generals are mostly ignored). Second, an isopathic prescription is combined with traditional prescribing. This is because this case was considered incurable allopathically and our previous experience has yielded similar poor results. The isopathic remedies add to the precision of action of the prescription.

Symptoms:

Chronic otitis externa of the right ear all his life, getting worse. There is a thick gluey brown discharge with a foul smell, but no pain. It is aggravated whenever water gets into his ear, particularly worse after swimming and during summer generally. This is particularly difficult since he likes to ocean surf. As a child he had grommets. He has had many courses of antibiotics and he uses herbal ear drops all of which have only afforded temporary relief. Acupuncture has no effect. When his ears are swabbed, cultures of *pseudomonas aeruginosa* and *staphylococcus aureus* (golden staph) are grown.

He is concerned because it is becoming worse with age.

He also has rashes under both arms and groin: a light brown colour which can itch. It appears to be one of the tineas or lichen skin diseases, though no diagnosis has been made.

Examination of the right ear shows a brown discharge, with a moist white film covering the tympanum.

In our experience infections such as these are stubborn and require pathological prescribing to cure them.

The patient was instructed to avoid all yeast foods and to absolutely avoid all water in the ear, since this provides a suitable environment for infection.

Prescription
1. Oral drops: *Pseudomonas + Aspergillus + Staph aureas 200* mixed with *Silicea 200*: One dose every second day.
2. Ear drops dispensed in pure ethanol: the above mix, minus the *Silicea*: One dose every second day (ie three doses per week) alternating with above drops. (Only use ethanol in the canal in adult patients when the drum is in tact and there are no eruptions in the canal).
3. *Psorinum 1M*: One dose per week on the day not taking the above drops.

Follow ups were monthly with steady improvement. Each month the potency of remedies 1 and 2 were raised: 1M, 10M, 20M, 50M. Silicea was kept at the same potency.

Psorinum was kept at the same potency until we reached 50M mixes, and was then increased to 10M. The patient experienced steady improvement until he was symptom free. It took almost four months for him to reach this stage. The rashes on his skin also improved dramatically but at the time of writing have not yet disappeared.

Another remedy will in all probability be required to cure his skin. Although the therapeutic protocol has had a beneficial effect on his skin lesions, it was his otitis externa for which he presented for treatment. Bearing this in mind, a homeopathic remedy to cover the whole case is not necessary (and indeed may not even exist).

Rationale for prescription:

We have never been able to cure pseudomonas of the external ear with traditional homeopathic prescribing. We therefore chose a combination of traditional remedies which exert a pathological influence on the ear canals, combined with isopathy.

Case 7: FM, female, age 56 - Hypothyroidism
This case illustrates the 'main remedy' approach chosen for the presenting condition; however there are also confirmatory individual symptoms (particulars and generals) for the same remedy. This offers a very certain prescription.

Symptoms:
o Exhaustion and nausea since four weeks: unable to carry out any physical activity without extreme and alarming exhaustion and weakness.
o Sleeps an average of eight hours, and feels well on waking.
o Irregular heart beat yet this is not evident on ECG.
o Long history of intolerance to alcohol, certain chemicals and foods: highly reactive to coffee, chocolate, cheese. Citrus may cause migraine with aura.
o Sensation of lump in throat.
o There is a fine tremor in her hands.
o She feels constantly jittery and wants to cry.

All medicals tests normal, yet she is taking the following medicines:
Cardizem (her blood pressure is actually normal, but erratic).
Hormone Replacement Therapy (HRT)
Folic acid
Iron supplement.
(She was also placed on an anti-arrhythmia medication shortly after seeing me).

History
Whooping cough.
Scarlet fever.
Tonsillectomy and adenoidectomy.

In this case there is no clear medical diagnosis despite a barrage of medical tests. It is not a case of Chronic Fatigue Syndrome, since in that syndrome one wakes tired even after a good sleep.
  She has some 'hysteric' type symptoms, with frequent sighing, jitters, and sense of lump in the throat. However, this does not really explain the sudden exhaustion and nausea. Despite normal TSH, we consider this a case of hypothyroidism, even though the disease has not produced an abnormal pathology report.
  Hypothyroidism, plus hysteric symptoms, strongly supports the choice of *Ignatia*. We decide, given the severity of her symptoms, to *Ignatia 200 and Thyroidinum 200* on alternate days (despite her specialist's dismissal of our diagnosis).
On her third visit her GP has organised a test for her free T4. After three months of our treatment the reading is 12.6 (10.0-23.0). Her General Practitioner commented it was likely that the T4 was below reference range when she commenced our treatment. We thus feel validated in our diagnosis of hypothyroidism (despite the skepticism of her specialist).

She improves well on this prescription for four months, until the symptom focus changes. The palpitations, exhaustion and 'hysteric' symptoms are much better, but she has a "heavy mind", with cloudy thinking and absent mindedness. These symptoms support a change in her prescription to another main remedy for hypothyroidism: *Gelsemium 200* alternated every second day. She improves on this remedy until all symptoms are cleared.

Rationale for prescription:
o *Ignatia* is a main remedy for hypothyroidism, plus she has several 'hysteric' symptoms found in that remedy: it is thus a confident prescription. It may not have been necessary (we will never know for sure) however *Thyroidinum 200* was alternated until she was stable.
o *Gelsemium 200:* was next chosen when her symptoms changed to *Gelsemium*-type symptoms. *Gelsemium* is also a main remedy in the treatment of hypothyroidism.

Case 8: EM, female, age 9 - Chronic Fatigue Syndrome

This case illustrates the choice of a 'main remedy' prescription where there are absolutely no individualising symptoms available. Normally the bane of homeopaths, these so-called 'one-sided' cases can respond well to the 'main remedy' which we have listed for each disease throughout this book.

Symptoms:
Headache, severe, daily since five months.
Body ache, especially knees and armpits.
Sore glands.
Anorexia and nausea.
Poor sleep: is woken constantly by the pain.
Wakes tired.
Photophobia.
Paresthesia: sensitive to the water touching her during her shower.
Slight constipation.
Abdominal pain.

There are no individualising symptoms of note: no modalities, significant food cravings, or peculiar mentals.
There are no discernable causations.
She does not want to attend the consultation or take our medicine. This is understandable considering she has had five months of medical tests, including a recent lumbar puncture, and has been placed on antidepressants because she is not eating. All pathology tests, including some exotic guesses such as toxoplasmosis and Ross River Virus, are negative.
Prior to her illness she appeared to be a normal child. No psychological factors are identified to suggest a reason for her symptom presentation.

This is a clear case of paediatric Chronic Fatigue Syndrome without a known cause. The unexplained pain, notably her headache, is the centre of the illness, since it prevents both sleep and appetite. The case remains serious, because the child cannot sleep or eat.

She responds immediately to *Calcarea phos 200* with steady improvement over the next eight weeks until she is symptom free. Eight weeks later she is back at school and functioning normally.

Rationale for prescription:

Calcarea phos 200: one dose every second day. This is the 'main remedy' for chronic headaches in children, as it is for chronic fatigue syndrome in children. With the absence of individual prescribing symptoms, or causation, this is the only remedy choice we could consider.

PART 6: PRACTICE FORMS

For Distribution to Patients

CHILDREN'S HOMEOPROPHYLAXIS PROGRAM

Name:——————————————————— is being protected against the following infectious diseases using high potency homeopathic remedies. Clinical studies over 200 years indicate that this program is non-toxic and comparably effective to conventional vaccines. The following chart indicates the current program status of the child and has been dated and signed by the parent on the administration of each remedy.

Age Recomm.	Age Given	Remedy	Potencies	Disease Relationship	Date Given	Given By
1 month		Pertussinum	200C, M, 10M	Whooping Cough		
2 months		Pneumococcinum	200C, M, 10M	Pneumococcal Disease		
3 months		Lathyrus sativus	200C, M, 10M	Poliomyelitis		
4 months		Hib Nosode	200C, M, 10M	Haemophilis Influenzae B		
5 months		Diphtherinum	200C, M, 10M	Diphtheria		
6 months		Tetanus toxinum	200C, M, 10M	Tetanus		
7 months		Meningococcinum	200C, M, 10M	Meningococcal Disease		
8 months		Morbillinum	200C, M, 10M	Measles		
9 months		Parotidinum	200C, M, 10M	Mumps		
10 months		Rubellinum	200C, M, 10M	Rubella (Germ. Measles)		
11 months		Varicellinum	200C, M, 10M	Chickenpox		
12 months		Hep B Nosode	200C, M, 10M	Hepatitis B		
1yr 1mth		Pertussinum	200C, M, 10M	Whooping Cough		
1yr 2mth		Pneumococcinum	200C, M, 10M	Pneumococcal Disease		
1yr 3mth		Lathyrus sativus	200C, M, 10M	Poliomyelitis		
1yr 4mth		Hib Nosode	200C, M, 10M	Haemophilis Influenzae B		
1yr 5mth		Diphtherinum	200C, M, 10M	Diphtheria		
1yr 6mth		Tetanus toxinum	200C, M, 10M	Tetanus		
1yr 7mth		Meningococcinum	200C, M, 10M	Meningococcal Disease		

Age	Age	Remedy	Potencies	Disease	Date	Given By
1yr 8mth		Morbillinum	200C, M, 10M	Measles		
1yr 9mth		Parotidinum	200C, M, 10M	Mumps		
1yr 10mth		Rubellinum	200C, M, 10M	Rubella (Germ. Measles)		
1yr 11mth		Varicellinum	200C, M, 10M	Chickenpox		
2 years		Hep B Nosode	200C, M, 10M	Hepatitis B		

☐ Kit A Remedies   ☐ Kit B Remedies

Note: Both children and adults can use this homeoprophylaxis (homeopathic immunisation) program. If the recipient is older than the "recommended age" on commencing the program, just enter their age in the "age given" column. The timing of all subsequent doses can then be calculated by adding the "recommended age" to their commencement age. See reverse for further instructions and guidelines.

Age Recomm.	Age Given	Remedy	Potencies	Disease Relationship	Date Given	Given By
3yr 1mth		Pertussinum	200C, M, 10M	Whooping Cough		
3yr 2mth		Pneumococcinum	200C, M, 10M	Pneumococcal Disease		
3yr 3mth		Lathyrus sativus	200C, M, 10M	Poliomyelitis		
3yr 4mth		Hib Nosode	200C, M, 10M	Haemophilis Influenzae B		
3yr 5mth		Diphtherinum	200C, M, 10M	Diphtheria		
3yr 6mth		Tetanus toxinum	200C, M, 10M	Tetanus		
3yr 7mth		Meningococcinum	200C, M, 10M	Meningococcal Disease		
3yr 8mth		Morbillinum	200C, M, 10M	Measles		
3yr 9mth		Parotidinum	200C, M, 10M	Mumps		
3yr 10mth		Rubellinum	200C, M, 10M	Rubella (Germ. Measles)		
3yr 11mth		Varicellinum	200C, M, 10M	Chickenpox		
4 years		Hep B Nosode	200C, M, 10M	Hepatitis B		
5yr 1mth		Pertussinum	200C, M, 10M	Whooping Cough		
5yr 2mth		Pneumococcinum	200C, M, 10M	Pneumococcal Disease		
5yr 3mth		Lathyrus sativus	200C, M, 10M	Poliomyelitis		
5yr 4mth		Hib Nosode	200C, M, 10M	Haemophilis Influenzae B		
5yr 5mth		Diphtherinum	200C, M, 10M	Diphtheria		

5yr 6mth		Tetanus toxinum	200C, M, 10M	Tetanus		
5yr 7mth		Meningococcinum	200C, M, 10M	Meningococcal Disease		
5yr 8mth		Morbillinum	200C, M, 10M	Measles		
5yr 9mth		Parotidinum	200C, M, 10M	Mumps		
5yr 10mth		Rubellinum	200C, M, 10M	Rubella (Germ. Measles)		
5yr 11mth		Varicellinum	200C, M, 10M	Chickenpox		
6 years		Hep B Nosode	200C, M, 10M	Hepatitis B		

© Fran Sheffield

General Instructions and Guidelines

1. For convenience it is suggested that each remedy be given by pilule in a series of three potencies (200C, M, and 10M) over a 24-hour period. To do this, give one 200C pilule in the morning, one M pilule that evening and one 10M pilule on the following morning. Alternatively, the pilules may be given one a day over three days or one a week over three weeks. Protection commences from the first dose. Place a line through each potency on the record as it is given.

2. The pilules must be given at least ½ hour either side of your child eating or drinking strong flavours (water is permitted) as flavours in the mouth can antidote the remedy.

3. Remedies do not have to be given in the listed order. Nor do all remedies have to be given. Remedies may be omitted or reordered to suit individual circumstances and preferences. Repetitions of each remedy should be at least 12 months apart.

4. For further information, please refer to the *Frequently Asked Questions* on the Do No Harm Initiative Inc website: www.d-n-h.org

A Homeoprophylaxis Consent Form is recommended in Australia for signing by both practitioner and patient. It can be downloaded at: www.aroh.com.au

Allergy Desensitising Protocol

Please follow this protocol. If you are unsure about any aspect, please contact the clinic.

Day		Medicine
1 3 5	} } }	Histaminum 10M
2 4 6	} } }	Allergen 200
7 9 11	} } }	Histaminum 50M
8 10 12	} } }	Allergen 30
13 15 17	} } }	Histaminum CM
14 16 18	} } }	Allergen 6

If there is a history of anaphylaxis, please do not ingest the allergen unless directed to do so and under proper supervision.

NB: you may develop 'allergy' type symptoms (eg sneezing, hives, etc) early in this protocol. This is a positive sign that the protocol is working and need not be regarded as a true allergic reaction. This reaction normally passes without intervention within 24 hours. If you are concerned about it please contact us.

PART 7: APPENDICES

Patient Handouts

DIETARY RECOMMENDATIONS FOR ASTHMA & ECZEMA

The most common problem parents tell us about their children's diet is that their children won't eat certain foods. As parents, we, not our children, are capable of knowing what is best for them.

"Let your food be your medicine and your medicine be your food"
-Hippocrates, the Greek Father of Modern Medicine

For optimum nutrition, health authorities recommend whole grains, 5 serves per day of fresh fruit and vegetables, (three veg & two fruit), daily protein such as meat, eggs and fish, plus small amount of fats and oils.

Foods which most often cause asthma & eczema symptoms are milk and milk products, wheat, yeast, eggs and peanuts.

When these foods are eliminated for up to 16 weeks children often show improvement of symptoms. The World Health Organisation (WHO) says that, in order to avoid allergies and digestive problems, babies should avoid being given wheat or dairy products until one year of age. Adults can improve when off dairy & wheat products. Buying a good allergy-free cookbook for alternative foods and recipes is really worthwhile

Food substitutes
Milk -> Goat's milk or soymilk.
There are many brands of soya milk available. Try the fresh one found in the supermarket fridge first. If your child must have milk, use biodynamic or organic whole, unhomogenised milks.

Yoghurt -> sheep's milk yoghurt, soya yoghurt & tofu dessert.
Buy good quality yoghurts with high acidophilus and bifidus content. Soya yoghurts, tofu desserts and sheep's milk yoghurts are available in 'non dairy' sections of supermarket fridges.

Cheese -> sheep & goat cheese.
Goat's cheese and sheep's cheese are easily available.

Wheat ->, Brown & white rice & their products, buckwheat, rye, soy & other flours, spelt flour, sago, tapioca, millet, quinoa.
It's common to have wheat in up to six meals and snacks every day. Once or twice daily is plenty. All bread should be 100% wholemeal – (check labels). Yeast free bread is available. The best supermarket brands to buy are Moores & Riga.

Meal substitutes
Breakfast – hot brown rice, fresh or stewed fruit, yoghurt (soy or dairy), porridge.
Lunch – the best time to have a sandwich. Include a green salad.

Dinner – meat or fish with green vegetables in addition to potato and corn. Apple crumble with a rolled oats topping is a healthy dessert.

Sandwiches & snacks - rice or corn crackers, hummus, fresh fruit, carrot sticks,

Baking –substitute wheat flour for flours mentioned above. Make pancakes, biscuits & cakes with a variety of flours.

Drinks

Water or much diluted fruit juice only. No soft drinks.

Fats & Oils

Use butter and/or olive oil mixes, but *not* margarine. Cook with olive oil bought in glass or tins, not in plastic. Fresh fish at least once weekly (if no seafood allergy) Nuts like walnuts, sunflower seeds, almonds & pepitas.

Foods to eliminate from the diet

All sweets, chips, cordials and other soft drinks. Nuttella is NOT healthy. Sugar has a depressant effect on the immune system. These foods are often high in fat and spoil children's appetites for healthy dinners. Takeaways should be kept to an absolute minimum.

Chemical content of foods –> Organic

The amount of chemicals in foods has increased enormously in the past 10-20 years, with little research done on the effects these have on human health and in particular, immunity. Children are particularly susceptible to pesticides, and chemical residues in foods which may trigger symptoms of inflammation. Organic food, particularly fruit and vegetables, are recommended.

Nutritional requirements for asthma & eczema

The aim of treatment is to reduce the inflammatory process in the lungs and skin, while enhancing general nutrition.

In the lungs, inflammation causes wheezing, mucus production and coughing. On the skin, redness, itching, flaking, oozing etc. Asthma and eczema generally respond well to an appropriate dietary regime.

Women taking the oral contraceptive pill need to take extra B group supplements.

Nutrients which help to reduce symptoms of asthma and eczema:

Vitamin B5 (Pantothenic Acid)

Alcohol, coffee, tea and stress increase the need for this vitamin. B5 helps the body to make cortisone and antibodies.

Source: Whole grains, green vegetables, avocado beans, egg yolk, milk, liver and oranges.

Vitamin B6

Helps metabolism of foods, especially fats and oils.

Source: Oatmeal, whole grains, legumes, tuna, salmon, mackerel, chicken, walnuts, meat and egg yolk.

Vitamin B12
Vitamin B12 helps to reduce the effects of toxins (chemicals from air and food). Maintains normal intestine and skin function.
Source: Liver, meat, oysters, sardines, salmon, herring, milk and eggs. Vegetarians need to take a supplement.

Vitamin C
Vitamin C is needed by the immune system due to its anti-viral and anti-bacterial action. It decreases fluid retention and helps to detoxify the body.
Source: Rosehips, black currants, citrus fruits, capsicum, cabbage, potatoes and pineapple. It is destroyed by processing and excessive cooking.

Vitamin A
Vitamin A is necessary for healthy skin and mucus membranes and resistance to infection.
Source: Animal and fish liver, kidneys, eggs, milk, dark leafy green and orange vegetables,

Vitamin E
Source: Egg yolk, wheat germ, nuts and vegetable oils.

Zinc
The majority of the Australian population is zinc deficient. Deficiency causes poor immunity, poor healing and skin problems.
Source: Oysters, liver, meat, seeds, green leafy vegetables and whole grains.

Magnesium
Magnesium is essential for the absorption of zinc and has a relaxant effect on the nervous system. Diets high in processed foods are often low in magnesium.
Source: Whole grains, green leafy vegetables, milk, nuts and soya beans.

Selenium
Needed for metabolism of essential fatty acids.
Source: Garlic, kelp, milk and eggs.

Essential fatty acids
Help to control inflammation and allergies.

DIETARY RECOMMENDATIONS FOR ACNE & PIMPLES

Aims of treatment
Reduce clogging and hardening of the pores -> Vitamin A & beta carotene, Vitamin E, selenium

Normalise bowel function - > fibre (vegetables & pulses)

Cleanse the liver -> Lemon juice in water on waking, 3 cups of dandelion coffee per day.

Balance testosterone -> zinc, B6

Normalise glucose tolerance -> chromium

Include
All fresh fruit & vegetables, cooked & raw. Carrot, beetroot, apple & celery juice with added ginger.

100% wholemeal grains, fresh fish

Meat and dairy products in small amounts

Beans, peas and lentils – in soups, and as spreads. (Hummus, split pea dip, three bean salad)

Oils – butter & olive oil in cooking and with food. Use spreads such as avocado, tahini, and hummus.

Avoid
Refined carbohydrates (white bread, cakes, biscuits, buns, pancakes etc)

Sugar and sweet foods – snack bars, chocolate.

Fried foods – bake, steam, or grill meals.

All homogenised oils: margarine, mayonnaise, butters made from oils, fried and barbequed foods

Which vitamins are in which foods? (Listed from highest to lowest amounts)

Vitamin A
Liver, red chilli peppers, dandelion greens, carrots, apricots, sweet potatoes, parsley, spinach, chives, squash, mangos

Vitamin E
Wheat germ, sunflower seeds, safflower oil, almonds, sesame, peanuts, olive oil. (Oils must be of the best quality)

Vitamin B6
Brewer's yeast (if tolerated) sunflower seeds, wheat germ, tuna, beef, chicken liver (organic) walnuts, salmon, trout.

Zinc
Oysters, ginger root, round steak, lamb chops, pecans, split peas, brazil nuts, beef liver (organic) egg yolk, whole wheat.

Chromium
Brewer's yeast (If tolerated) calf liver, whole wheat or rye bread. These are all high in the Glucose Tolerance Factor.

Selenium
Butter, smoked herring, wheat germ, brazil nuts, apple cider vinegar, barley, wholemeal bread, oats, crab, oysters, milk.

A high dose multi vitamin and mineral supplement is recommended. This ensures adequate doses of the minerals zinc and selenium, which are lacking in Australian soils and therefore the food.
Foods should be organic where possible, to avoid consumption of chemicals, pesticide residues and antibiotics.

PREVENTING EAR INFECTIONS

Elements that help keep children healthy so they avoid problems like ear infections:

o Good health

o Stimulating the body's healing response

o Protecting from triggers and treating early symptoms

o Treating underlying problems which lead to ear infections (colds, tonsillitis, and allergies).

Good health
The best way to achieve good health in a child is through proper nutrition and limiting exposure to other coughs and colds. Frequent hand washing for children is recommended.

To stimulate the body's healing response
o Add extra nutrition, in the form of Vitamin C or kiddy vitamins

o Give herbs like Echinacea

o Use Homeopathic medicines where needed

o Fevers also stimulate immune activity. Only use paracetamol or other antipyretics when the fever is above 39°C

o Ensure your child is having enough sleep.

Antibiotics should be used as a last resort, not the first. Many studies indicate that antibiotics are given when the ear infection is viral and that 'watching and waiting' can give similar results.

 Helping the immune system: *Over 80% of immune activity takes place in the bowel, - yes, the bowel, in special lymphatic tissue called Peyer's patches. Antibiotics can disrupt the immune activity in the bowel and weaken the immune response for the next exposure to a bacteria or virus.*

Environment
Keep children's ears covered in cold weather with a woollen had pulled down well over the ears. Snow skiing head bands work really well.

Diet

Many children's ear infections lessen or stop completely when they are on a dairy-free and low wheat diet. Substitute cow's milk for goat's milk & use sheep's milk yoghurt. Rice crackers and rice cakes make great snacks. Cook rice instead of pasta for a few meals per week.

Treating early symptoms

Using homeopathic medicines to treat the early symptoms of colds and sore throats often avoids an ear infection developing. When used effectively, the cold or sore throat lasts a shorter time, symptoms are mild and they don't develop into any other illness, like an ear infection.

Treating underlying problems

When children do not respond to the usual simple measures for their illness and repeatedly become sick, the cause needs to be found. It could be that the problem runs in the family; there is an allergy, poor absorption of nutrients or poor resistance to infections. These children need individualised homeopathic treatment to address these problems. *The best time to treat a child is during times when they are not suffering from health problems like colds and ear infections.* This is when preventative treatment can take place.

Other therapies

- Osteopathic and chiropractic treatment can help some children who get frequent ear infections.
- Herbal medicines may also be helpful.

TREATING EARLY SYMPTOMS IN EAR INFECTIONS

Clear runny nose
When a clear runny nose starts, give five drops of *PCIP* (*Kali mur & Ferrum phos*) every two to four hours, depending on the severity of symptoms

Thick, coloured runny nose
If nose mucus becomes coloured quickly, use *Pulsatilla 30* two to three times daily.

Exposure to cold
If an earache comes on quickly after being exposed to a cold dry wind, give *Aconite 4x* every half hour until the pain settles.

Teething
If symptoms come as a result of teething, give *Chamomilla 30* either every half hour until settled, or three times daily during teething.

If tonsillitis comes before an ear infection, *Hepar sulph 200* given twice daily reduces the tonsillitis and may prevent the ear infection developing.

Fevers
For fevers below 38.5°C, give either *PCIP (Kali mur & Ferrum phos*) every half hour, or *Ferrum Phos 30* every 30 minutes.

Fever coming on suddenly, the child is lethargic; the ear is red, give *Belladonna 200* every 1/2-hour until symptoms settle. Remember, fevers help your child's immune system fight the problem.

High fever, child's face looks red, give *Belladonna 200*. If child is restless, give *Aconite 200*.

Suspected Ear Infection
Early stages of ear infections use 'ABC' (*Aconite, Belladonna & Chamomilla*) every one to two hours, depending on severity of symptoms

IMPORTANT NOTE:
The above remedies are a GENERAL guide to common first aid situations only and are *NOT SUITABLE FOR ONGOING CONDITIONS.*
- They do NOT substitute professional medical care.
- If the condition you are treating is not responding, contact your health professional.

SOURCES OF CALCIUM

*This list is a **general guide only** to calcium containing foods and does not include every calcium containing food. **Bold type indicates rich calcium sources.***

Food	Quantity	mgs	Food	Quantity	mgs
Almonds	1 cup	332	Lentils, cooked	1 cup	50
Apricots	1 cup	87			
			Melon- honeydew	150mgs	21
Barley	1cup cooked	68	**Milk whole**	**1 cup**	**291**
Beans black	**1 cup**	**270**	Milk, soy	1 cup	47
Beans green	1cup	62	Millet, cooked	1 cup	45
Beans, pinto	1 cup	**357**			
Beans, kidney	1 cup	70	Nectarine	1 raw	23
Beans, soy	1 cup	131			
Beef	500g	34 -54	Orange	1	54
Beet greens raw	100mgs	119			
Beet greens cooked	1 cup	131	Paw paw	1/2 medium	30
Brazil nuts	1 cup	260	Peaches dried	1 cup	77
Bread, wholemeal	1 slice	63	Pears dried	1 cup	63
Broccoli	**1 x 5inch**	**136**	Pecan pie	1 slice	75
Butter	**piece**	45	Potato	1 cup	36
	1 TBSP		Prunes	1 cup	90
Cabbage		64	Pumpkin pie	1 slice	76
Carob powder	1 cup cooked	17			
Carrots	1 tsp	51	Raisins	1 cup	102
Cauliflower	1 cup cooked	26	**Rhubarb**	**1 cup**	**117**
Cherries	1 cup cooked	34	Rice, brown	1 cup	18
Chick peas	1 cup fresh	**300**			
Cornflakes	**1 cup**	30	**SEAWEEDS**		
	1 cup		**Arame**	**100g**	**1000**
Dates		59	**Kelp**	**100g**	**1093**
	10 medium		**Hijiki**	**100g**	**1400**
Eggs		22/31	**Kombu**	**100g**	**800**
	1 small/large		**Nori**	**100g**	**260**
		35	**Wakame**	**100g**	**1300**
Figs raw	2 large	126			
Figs dried	5 medium		Sesame seeds	1 cup	165
FISH		258	Sunflower seeds	1 cup	174
Herring	500g	**388**			
Mackerel, tinned	**1 cup**	426	Tangerine	1	34
Oysters fresh	500g	**570**	Tofu	100g	42
Salmon tinned	**1 cup**	124	Tortilla	6" diameter	60
Sardines	1 cup	286	**Walnuts**	**1 cup**	**282**
Shrimp	500g		Wheat germ	1 cup	72
		24			
Grapes	1 cup				

REFERENCES: *Nutrition Almanac 1989 McGraw Hill Book Co*
Nutrients in Profile Henry Osieki Bioconcepts Publishing 2nd Edn

CORTISONE CREAMS AND PUFFERS

There is no doubt that cortisone creams and puffers often give good control of asthma & eczema symptoms. They do come with their side effects though. Due to its side effects, cortisone should be used only as a last resort, having first tried less invasive treatments. When considering giving cortisone preparations, the condition needs to be severe enough to warrant the potential loss in bone density in men and women, and growth in children. These side effects may be offset by taking vitamin and mineral supplements.

Cortisone *is* effective for reducing inflammation, in lungs or skin.
The body naturally produces cortisone. In allergic patients cortisone production from the adrenal glands is not enough to overcome symptoms.
Because cortisone does not treat the cause, the patient has control of symptoms only while on medication.
When cortisone creams are suddenly stopped being used in a skin disease, there can be a 'rebound' effect. Skin inflammation can return with a vengeance! If this coincides with the homeopathic treatment, it is often mistaken for the new, treatment either not working or making the problem worse.
Stopping puffers and oral cortisone medication must be done gradually, under careful supervision.
Side effects may be offset by taking vitamin & mineral supplements

One of the best natural anti-inflammatory treatments (aside from finding the cause of the problem) is to change oils in the diet. Depending on the severity of the condition:

Reduce or eliminate red meat from the diet
Eat fresh, deep-sea fish as often as possible
Take an oil supplement.

Oil Supplements
Omega 3 oils
Fish oils
Cod liver oil
Flaxseed, or linseed oil
Borage oil.
Food sources of oil: Fresh fish, nuts (almonds, walnuts, not peanuts), sunflower seeds, pumpkin seeds, pepitas.

INSTRUCTIONS WHILE TAKING HOMEOPATHIC MEDICINE

Homeopathic medicines are easily antidoted. For best results, please follow these instructions:

o *Take your drops or pilules 15-30 minutes away from eating, drinking and brushing your teeth, as homeopathic medicines are absorbed through the lining of your mouth (and not your stomach)*

o *Store medicines in a cool, dark, dry place (not the fridge) and keep away from sunlight, heat and strong smells like perfumes, Vicks, kitchen spices, eucalyptus oil and liniments.*

o *Avoid touching the pilules with fingers or the bottle dropper with your mouth, and hold the medicine under your tongue for ten seconds or so before swallowing.*

o *Do not apply Vicks, eucalyptus oil or other strong smelling substances like perfumes to your child, or yourself, during homeopathic treatment.*

Homeopathic Medicines are safe for children and pregnant women to take, as there are no toxic side effects.

If your symptoms change while on homeopathic treatment and you are concerned about what to do next, please contact us.

REMEMBER TO FOLLOW DOSAGE INSTRUCTIONS CAREFULLY

Practitioner stamp:

WHAT TO EXPECT WHILE ON HOMEOPATHIC MEDICINE

Our aim is for you to become symptom free as quickly as possible.
Taking homeopathic medicine is different from taking medical drugs, which are often taken long-term to keep control of symptoms.
Our approach is to remove the cause of your health problem. This takes more time and effort than simply getting symptomatic relief. Therefore, a series of treatments is usually necessary to remove long-term symptoms, rather than a single visit for medicine to remove only the most troublesome symptoms.
Generally speaking, the longer you have had a condition, the longer it takes to remove all your symptoms.

To gain the most from your treatments:

o When you experience a change in your symptoms after taking your first prescription and it is more than a week before your next appointment, please contact us for further instructions.

o To *maintain* improvement after a first visit, follow up care is essential.

o If you do not experience any changes in your symptoms after taking your first prescription and you still have troublesome symptoms, let us know and we can move your appointment forward. Your dosage or medicine will probably be changed at this next appointment. Long-term health problems require time and skill to successfully treat.

Remember, homeopathic medicines have been used safely and effectively for over 200 years for a wide range of health problems in adults and children. If you have any queries about homeopathy and how it works, please phone us for more information.

Practitioner stamp:

SALICYLATE CONTENT OF FOODS

Food Type	Negligible	Low	Moderate	High	Very High
FRUIT	Cavendish bananas, Peeled pears.	Golden Delicious apples, pawpaw, pomegranate	Custard apple, Figs, lemon, loquats, mango, pear (unpeeled), persimmon, Red Delicious apple, rhubarb, tamarillo.	Avocado, Granny Smith apple, grapefruit, Jonathon apple, kiwi fruit, lychee, mandarin, mulberry, nectarine, passion fruit, peach, tangelo, watermelon.	Apricot, blackberry, black currant, blueberry, boysenberry, cherry, cranberry, currants, dates, grape, guava, loganberry, plum, pineapple, prune, raisins, red currant, rock melon, strawberry, sultana.
VEGETABLES	Bamboo shoots, dried beans, cabbage, celery, brown & red lentils, lettuce, dried peas, peeled potato, swede.	Brussels sprouts, chives, choko, green beans, green peas, leeks, mung bean sprouts, red cabbage, shallots.	Asparagus, beetroot, broccoli, carrot, cauliflower, marrow, mushroom, onion, parsnip, pumpkin spinach, sweet corn, sweet potato, turnip.	Alfalfa sprouts, broad beans, cucumber, eggplant, watercress.	Capsicum, champignon, chicory, gherkin, endive, hot pepper, tomato & its products, olive, radish, zucchini.
NUTS & SEEDS	Poppy seed	Cashews	Brazil nut, coconut, hazelnut, macadamias, peanut, pecans, pine nut, pistachio, sesame seeds, sunflower seeds, walnuts.		Almonds, water chestnuts.
SWEETS	Cocoa, carob, maple syrup, maple sugar.	Caramels, golden syrup.	Molasses		Honey, licorice, peppermints.
HERBS & SPICES		Garlic, malt vinegar, parsley, saffron, soy sauce, tandoori, vanilla.		Allspice, bay leaf, black pepper, caraway, cardamom, cinnamon, cloves, ginger, nutmeg, pimento, white pepper, white vinegar.	Aniseed, canella, cayenne, cumin, curry, dill, five spice, garam masala, marmite, mint, mixed herbs, mustard, oregano, paprika, rosemary, sage, tarragon, thyme, turmeric, vegemite, Worcester sauce.
BEVERAGES	**INSTANT COFFEES** Andronicus, Pablo, Decaff. **Other:** Aktivite, Milo, Oval tine. **Alcohol:** Gin, whiskey, vodka.	**INSTANT COFFEES** Harris, Bushells Instant & Turkish, Robert Timms. Chamomile tea. **Other:** Ecco, Bambu, dandelion	**INSTANT COFFEES:** Harris mocha, International Roast, Nescafe. **TEAS** decaffeinated, fruit, rosehip. **Cereal coffees:** Reform. **Other:** Rosehip syrup, fruit juice, coke. **Alcohol:** Brandy, beer, cider, sherry.		**TEA:** All brands, peppermint **Cereal coffee:** Nature's Cuppa **Alcohol:** Liqueur, port, rum, wine.

ALLOPATHIC TREATMENTS FOR ASTHMA & THEIR SIDE EFFECTS

Bronchodilators (Relievers)

B2 adrenoceptors agonists	Brand name	Common side effects
Salbutamol [Action: stimulates lung receptors that are affected by adrenaline-like substances.]	Ventolin, Asmol, Airomir, Respolin	Palpitations, muscle tremor, vasodilation (feeling warm), possible hypotension and headache. Hyperactivity. Weaken lungs & heart. Death rate from asthma higher in those taking bronchodilators.
Terbutaline	Bricanyl	Ditto
Fenoterol	Berotec	[This drug has caused fatalities and is now withdrawn.]
Salmeterol	Serevent, Optrol	Ditto
Eformoterol	Foradile, Oxis	Ditto
Xanthine drugs		
Theophylline	Theo-dur, Austyn, Nuelin, Brondecon, Somophyllin	Increased heart rate, arrhythmia, CNS disturbance (anxiety, tremor, insomnia), GIT disturbance (anorexia, nausea & vomiting. Hyperactivity.
Theobromine	Coffee, tea, cola, cocoa, chocolate	Palpitations, insomnia
Muscarinic-receptor antagonists		
Ipratropium	Atrovent, ipratrin	Dry mouth, constipation, urine retention.

Anti-inflammatory agents (preventers)

Glucocorticoids	Brand name	Side effects
Beclomethasone	Becotide, Becloforte, Respocort	Oral thrush. Osteoporosis, impaired growth in children, thinning skin; compromised immunity. Allergic reactions. Thrombosis. Oedema. Gastric ulcer. Weight gain. Nausea. Convulsions. Endocrine disorders eg diabetes, cushingoid state. Menstrual disorders. Psychosis. Skin lesions. Cataracts. Exophthalmus.
Budesonide	Pulmicort,	Ditto
Fluticasone	Flixotide, Seretide	Ditto
Prednisolone (oral)	Delta-cortef, Panaf Cortelone	
Methylprednisolone (oral)	Medrol	Ditto
Hydrocortisone (intravenous)	Hysone, Nordicort	Ditto
Cromoglycate or nedocromil	Intal, Tilade (children)	cough
Leukotriene antagonists	Singulair, Accolagte	Headache, nausea

Bibliography

- Banerji, Dr Parimal, *Advanced Homeopathy and its Materia Medica*, Advanced Thinkers, Calcutta, Vols 1-3,1986-1995 plus lectures, conference notes and booklets.
- Boericke, Dr William, *Pocket Manual of Homeopathic Materia Medica*, 9th ed. revised, B Jain, New Delhi, 1991.
- Elmiger, Dr Jean, *Rediscovering Real Medicine,* Vega, London, 2001
- Foubister, Dr Donald, *Tutorials in Homeopathy*, Beaconsfield Publishers, Bucks, 1989.
- Gamble, J, *Mastering homeopathy 2: The Treatment of Irritable Bowel Syndrome,* Karuna publishing, 2006
- Gamble, j & Hermiston N, *Treat Your Child yourself,* Karuna Publishing, 2007
- Gascoigne, Dr Stephen, *The Clinical Medicine Guide*, *A Holistic Perspective*, Jigme Press, Co Cork, Ireland.
- Golden, Isaac, *Homeoprophylaxis - A Fifteen Year Clinical Study: A Statistical Review of the Efficacy and the Safety of Long-term Homeoprophylaxis.* 2004. ISBN 0 9578 726 3 1. www.users.connect.com.au/~homstudy/
- Hahnemann, Dr Samuel, *Organon of Medicine,* 5th ed (1833) trans. Dudgeon, B Jain, Delhi.
- Harris, Kathy, *Managing Menopause Naturally: A Comprehensive Clinician's Manual*, Kathy Harris Holistic Healing, Sydney 2002. ISBN 0 9581816 0 8.
- Herscu, Paul, *The Homeopathic Treatment of Children,* North Atlantic Books, Berkeley, CA, 1991.
- Julian, Dr O A, *Materia Medica of New Homoeopathic Remedies*, Beaconsfield Publishers, Bucks, UK, 1979.
- Lockie, Dr Andrew, *The Family Guide to Homeopathy,* Hamish Hamilton, London, 1989.
- Murphy, Robin, *Homeopathic Medical Repertory*, 1st ed, Hahnemann Academy of North America, 1993.
- Paterson, Dr J, *The Bowel Nosodes,* B Jain, New Delhi, 1988.
- Sheppard, Dorothy, *Homeopathy in Epidemic Diseases,* Health Science Press, UK, 1978.
- Smits, Dr Tinus, lecture presentations. Website: www.tinussmits.com/english/
- Tumminello, Peter, *The Child's Mind and Behaviour*, 2nd ed, The Medical Way, Sydney, 1991. ISBN 0-646-41172-1.
- Vermeulen, Frans, *Concordant Materia Medica,* Merlijn Publishers, Naarlem, 1994.

Useful Resources

Australian Homeopathic Association: www.homeopathyoz.org
Recent news, help with finding a practitioner in Australia.

Australian Register of Homeopaths: www.aroh.com.au
The registration board for homeopaths in Australia.

Homeopathy Clinic: For further health information and client questionnaires.
www.homeopathyworks.com.au

Index

All references are to paragraph numbers
'ff' = 'and following paragraphs'

All references are to paragraph numbers
'ff' = 'and following paragraphs'

All references are to paragraph numbers
'ff' = 'and following paragraphs'

All references are to paragraph numbers
'ff' = 'and following paragraphs'

Acknowledgements

First, I wish to acknowledge the work of Dr Parimal Banerji of Calcutta. Dr Banerji's breadth of knowledge of materia medica, his empirical research to determine the most efficacious potencies, and to classify particular symptom groupings, have made an enormous contribution to our profession. While this book does not purport to represent his work, my study with the doctor and his associates in Calcutta has certainly reframed the way I look at clinical practice.

Alan Jones' methods, particularly the use of nosodes and isopathy, are also acknowledged.

I have learned much from many colleagues: a few of whom are David Levy, Ken D'Aran, Patricia Janssen, Peter Tumminello and John Maitland. Thank you to Tina Mullholland for her enthusiastic graphic cover design and to Dr Michael Tomlinson for early draft comments. A special thank you to Patricia Janssen for her detailed reading and comments of the first draft.

My greatest acknowledgement goes to Nyema Hermiston, not only for her contribution of the patient handouts in this book, but for her ongoing encouragement, our earnest discussions, and her creative feedback, without which this book would not have manifested.

Titles by Jon Gamble, available from Karuna Publishing:

Mastering Homeopathy 2: The Treatment of Irritable Bowel Syndrome (2006)

Mastering Homeopathy 3: Obstacles to Cure (with Nyema Hermiston)(scheduled for 2010)

Treat Your Child yourself: A Parent's Guide to Drug-Free Solutions for Common Complaints (with Nyema Hermiston) (2007)

These titles may be purchased online at www.homeopathyworks.com.au or at your homeopathic book stockist.

www.ingramcontent.com/pod-product-compliance
Lightning Source LLC
LaVergne TN
LVHW020218110325
805655LV00009B/481

*9 7 8 0 9 7 5 2 4 7 3 0 3 *